About the Author

Danièle Ryman was born in Cahors, France, and at the age of twenty discovered her vocation when she met the pioneer of aromatherapy, Marguerite Maury. After years of training, she came to Britain to run the Marguerite Maury Clinic in London. She has been practising for twenty-one years and specialises in skin problems. A regular participant in *Cosmopolitan*'s Health Workshops, Danièle has also contributed to several alternative health books and broadcasts frequently on television.

The Aromatherapy Handbook

The Secret Healing Power of Essential Oils

Danièle Ryman

THE C. W. DANIEL COMPANY LIMITED
SAFFRON WALDEN

First published in Great Britain 1984
by Century Publishing Co. Ltd,
Portland House,
12-13 Greek St, London W1V 5LE

Reprinted 1989 by The C. W. Daniel Company Limited,
1 Church Path
Saffron Walden
Essex
England

Second Impression July 1989
Third Impression August 1990

ISBN 0-85207-215-5

Produced by Ennisfield Print & Design, London

Contents

Dedication

In memory of Marguerite Maury

NOTE

Aromatherapy is a form of complementary medicine and I would advise any patients under medication not to stop their treatment in order to try a formulation or suggestion without first consulting their doctors.

Introduction

This aromatherapy self-help handbook is dedicated to women in particular. It has been written because there is a need for information on this alternative form of medicine – and also because of constant nagging from my patients to record the advice given to them over twenty-one years!

Aromatherapy has been a way of life for me since the very first day of my life. The room in which I was born was filled with peach blossom and lilac, and I was later told by my grandmother that it was customary to welcome a baby in this manner, as its first breath of fresh air should be vivified through the scent of flowers. Thereafter, throughout my youth, with my family I practised the therapy without ever being conscious of its name. We massaged oils on our bodies when tired, took tisanes for insomnia and digestive upsets, inhaled the essential oils of plants when we suffered from bronchitis, colds and flu, and even used aromatic substances in cooking to help digestion. It was not unusual either to go on walks in the pine forests to breathe the pine scent, believed to be a preventative against tuberculosis.

It was Marguerite Maury, the pioneer of aromatherapy, whom I met in Paris when I was twenty, who made me aware that I had been practising it all my life. It was she who also convinced me that it could be taken seriously, and that I would be able to express my need to treat and heal people through it. So my life took this direction and I left the Beaux Arts, where I had been studying art, and went to work under her guidance until she died in 1968.

After her death I carried on her work and research. Later I widened its scope to include the sense of smell with aromatherapy itself, as I felt this had always been neglected because of our culture's visual bias. When I began delving into the subject, I discovered that this had not always been the case. In the past, people had been far more aware of the sense of smell and the therapeutic function of smell.

The purpose of this book is to make people realise that this form of alternative medicine is open to all to practise and can bring nature back into urban lives through a 'rainbow' of scents. After all, we should not forget what Hippocrates, the father of medicine, said: 'The way to health is to have an aromatic bath and scented massage every day.'

Danièle Ryman, January 1984

CHAPTER ONE

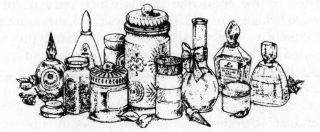

The Sense of Smell

The sense of smell seems sadly neglected today, whilst the senses of vision and hearing are increasingly relied upon for giving information about the environment in which we live. Historically, the sense of smell was one of the most potent constituents of behaviour and indeed of survival, but nowadays most of us are not even aware that the sense of smell is one of the subtlest means of communication we possess, nor that it is one of the earliest means by which we form a bond with our new world. When a baby is born, the first thing he does is to take a deep breath, inhaling the different odours in the air and, because his eyesight is poor, he uses his sense of smell to recognise his mother and the security she represents for him. To primitive men and women, the sense of smell was as important as it is still for many animals, and it is only so-called 'civilisation' that has made us neglect its influence.

PHEROMONES

For humans, like animals, produce odoriferous substances called *pheromones* (the name comes from the Greek *pherein*, to carry, and *hormon*, to excite), which are used to identify, attract, and – in animals – to mark territory.

Human pheromones are chemically similar to the hormones secreted by the endocrine glands which circulate in the blood to bring about all kinds of physical changes, but they are actually manufactured by the apocrine glands (not to be confused with those which produce sebum and sweat, found lying just beneath the skin, mostly around the breasts, under the arms, and in the anal and genital areas). We all emit pheromones which radiate into the air around us and are detected by other people – usually totally oblivious to the influence they may be having upon them – and by animals too.

To animals, the pheromones they emit act as a kind of language whereby they communicate with one another. Dogs, cats of all kinds, and many other animals leave scents to pass on messages about territory, destination, sex, etc. A hunted fox with a pack of hounds following his scent, for instance, will backtrack several times across a river to muffle the aroma of his trail, and will always search for a flock of sheep or other animals with whom he can mingle, thus losing his smell identity. Primitive tribesmen smeared their skins with animal scents in an attempt to camouflage their own phoromones and prevent them being detected by enemies, an idea probably suggested by their observations of the animal world.

Indeed, studying the habits of ancient or primitive peoples lends much support to the notion that they used their sense of smell to a much greater extent than it is used today, to its full potential indeed, in tandem with the senses of sight, sound and touch. Primitive man would sniff the ground to find out whether other peoples had passed that way – which makes sense, as several apocrine glands are found on the soles of the feet and pheromone molecules are known to linger on the soil for as long as fifteen days. American Indians did this until comparatively recently, and they were also known to be able to smell the odour of a dead man's body up to ten miles away.

Perhaps the reason we have moved away from using our sense of smell is because we associate sniffing with animal behaviour, seeing it as a primitive function that civilised man should leave behind him if he wishes to be superior in the animal kingdom. Standing on two feet probably had something to do with it too. But whatever the reason, we are now having to rediscover the roles that pheromones play in our lives, and much of the evidence which suggests that smells act as messengers and alter our behaviour patterns comes from studies of animals.

In animals, the other important purpose of pheromones lies in sexual attraction – most obvious in the Emperor moth, whose mate can be attracted by smell from several miles away – and the fact that different animals produce their own variety of pheromones is obviously influential in ensuring the survival and healthy proliferation of the species. But research suggests that men and women too are sexually responsive to the pheromones that each emits. (Generally speaking, the pheromones produced by men have a musky aroma whereas women's, although similar, are usually subtler and perhaps rather sweeter.)

The quality of those produced by a woman varies throughout her monthly cycle, and a man is most receptive and attracted to her smells at the time of ovulation. A woman's sensitivity to a man's pheromones also soars and plummets periodically due to the constant fluctations in her sex hormones. A man in New Guinea, for instance, will unashamedly waft a handkerchief that has been tucked in his armpit under the nostrils of his partner to arouse her to passion after the last dance. And, although not directly linked with sexual attraction, it is well known that a woman's sense of smell becomes dulled from about two days after conception until about the third month: if this phenomenon could be used to confirm pregnancy, it would be considerably more pleasant than some of the medical tests currently performed!

As the quality of pheromones we produce can be influenced by the fluctations of hormones within the body, so they can also change when we are frightened. It is a literary cliché, but it *is* possible to detect fear in each other through the sense of smell. Animals certainly change their pheromones when attacked or frightened: when an ant's nest, for instance, is invaded by an intruder some of the ants secrete a different quality of pheromone which is perceived by the others and they will then rally together to ward off their undesirable visitor. And animals can detect this emotion in humans: it is how a horse or dog can sense when you are nervous, and it may also help to explain why in times of war people tend to become much closer and more protective towards one another.

In fact, your sense of smell can protect you from all kinds of danger, and in my experience it can even save your life. Whilst asleep, most human senses are dulled, but the olfactory sense retains its acuity for all twenty-four hours of the day and night. This was invaluable to the survival of primitive man for while he rested, exposed to the elements, he could be assured of being able to detect the presence of a threatening stranger or animal. Nowadays, although we can lock doors for safety, the ability to detect unusual obtrusive odour is still a very precious asset. Twice my sense of smell has warned me of the presence of fire, waking me during the night in time to let me save the lives of my family and myself. During waking hours, too, it can tell of the presence of a gas leak or poisonous fumes, allowing you to react in time to escape from the impending danger.

Interestingly, the sense of smell is very often deadened when you are unwell, not only if you have a cold or flu, but also if you have another illness which does not necessarily interfere with the nasal passages, and we should always be aware of this.

THE SENSE OF SMELL AND THE PSYCHE

What do different aromas consist of, and how do they work to have such profound effects on behaviour, mood and functioning of the body?

We usually refer to a smell as something that is rather offensive, whereas an odour is neutral, neither particularly pleasant or unpleasant, and a scent is applied to perfume or the trail left by an animal. However, they are really all the same thing, odoriferous substances which consist of volatile molecules that can pass through air and water. The study or science of smell is technically called 'osmology' (from the Greek *osme*, smell), and odoriferous substances or smells are known as osmyls. Unlike light and sound, scientists have not quantified smell into measurable units, perhaps because the mechanism of smell perception still remains rather a mystery.

The molecules of an odour are perceived by a bundle of highly sensitive nerve cells located on the membranes lining the nasal passages (nostrils). These nerve cells make up the organ of olfaction which in humans is no larger in size than a thumb print, but in animals can be ten to thousands of times larger, which helps to explain why their sense of smell is far more developed than ours. Nevertheless, our sense of smell is 10,000 times more sensitive than that of taste, and as each of the nerves in the nose is a tiny branch of the brain, information about a certain smell is relayed incredibly quickly, whereas the detection of taste, sound, and touch is far less direct.

During our lifetime the degree to which we use our sense of smell changes. Babies rely heavily on the olfactory organ to help them seek nourishment for they can detect the pheromones a mother secretes from her breasts as well as the sweet odour of her milk. In early childhood too we react spontaneously to different smells, and studies suggest that children with a sharp sense of smell are often the most intelligent. However, children are unable naturally to discriminate between a good smell and a bad one, and pick up most of their notions as to which smells are acceptable and which are nasty from parents or schoolfriends.

Research has shown, however, that young children are highly attracted to the smell of strawberries and vanilla. To my disgust I discovered that many manufacturers have capitalised on this by scenting the rubber with which children's dolls are made with artificial strawberry essence. I strongly suspect that the current fashion of scenting things like erasers and teeshirts with imitation essences could lead ultimately to much more dangerous tendencies like glue sniffing. Artificial odours and flavourings are even added to baby foods, creating the illusion that pears or apples are present in much greater abundance than they actually are.

Between the ages of ten and eighteen, children develop a liking for the fragrances of orange and musk as well as strawberries and vanilla, and it is not until the twenties that the sense of smell becomes rather more sophisticated, when individual preferences and dislikes for different odours are displayed. So even when two fragrances are generally accepted as being pleasant – say carnation and rose – a person may show a preference for one and actively dislike the other. This individuality plays an important role in determining the people to whom we are attracted, the kind of environment we feel happiest in, the flowers we would choose for the home and so on. (It is interesting to note that men are attracted to more complex mixes of spicy and floral fragrances whereas women tend to prefer the simple, single ones.)

Another intriguing aspect of smells or aromas is their ability to evoke memories – not just visual images of past happenings, but also the emotions felt at that time. I will always remember the smell of my mother's perfume, Rose of Rochas. It still has a calming and comforting influence on me, as I associate it with her coming upstairs to kiss us goodnight. In the same way, the smell of Gitanes tobacco reminds me of my father for it used to impregnate his hair, skin and clothes, and in its presence I feel secure and protected.

Why don't you experiment yourself with memories by imagining different smells? Shut your eyes and remember the first time you went to the seaside. Concentrate on the smell of the salt and seaweed – this should make you feel excited and happy. Conjure up the smell of the country, of farms, chickens and cows, of fields of corn and wheat, the smell of pine forests. Travel back in time and remember your first day at school, and you will probably sense a feeling of anticipation mixed with fear and excitement as you recall the smell of wooden desks and blackboards. Remember your first love and the flowers he may perhaps have given you. Such smells invariably evoke pleasurable sensations. Poets and writers have often gained inspiration from different scents: Proust, when he lived in Paris, for example, would travel 100 kilometres to Normandy to inhale the apple blossom. It is also interesting to note that different fragrances often feature strongly when there is mention of love in novels or poems.

To me a sharp and discriminating sense of smell is an incredibly valuable possession and I am very lucky to have been born with one. When I was young I could recognise my mother's friends by the trail of scent they would leave in the corridors. I felt very wary of one of them and I'm sure she probably had a hostile smell although I didn't understand this at the time. It was not until several years later that I learned from my mother that she had one day found her friend secretly drinking some of my milk ration (for it was during the war), and topping it up with water. Strangely enough, we have a saying in French *'Je ne peux pas le sentir'* which literally translated means 'I can't smell him', meaning

'I don't trust or like him'. This is probably a residual memory of when we would have used our sense of smell to determine whether we were attracted or repelled by another person's pheromones.

THE SENSE OF SMELL NOWADAYS

It seems a shame to me that we have become obsessed with washing away the very smells that attract other people to us – the pheromones – keeping them at bay by using deodorants and replacing them with perfumes. I'm sure that it is because we are continually told, via the media, that the secretions we produce smell unpleasant, and we have been instilled with a fear of uncleanliness should we allow them to linger. Of course, this is a terrible distortion of the truth, firstly because within a matter of half an hour they will have been replaced again, and secondly because there is nothing unclean or unpleasant about our pheromones. In fact they are very attractive, and for this reason perfumers use extracts of animal glands such as civet, ambergris and musk in their creations, as they are known to appeal to our sense of smell due to their similarity in nature to our own secretions. Indeed, I believe that the eccentric painter Salvador Dali used to rub male goats' faeces into his moustache before going out for the evening. As he was considered incredibly attractive to and successful with women, this unusual facet of his nocturnal preparations would seem to bear this point out!

Not only do I find the idea perpetrated by the perfume and scent manufacturers that we should replace our own natural fragrances with imitations one of bad taste, I also know it can be harmful. Because the raw materials are incredibly expensive, synthetic substitutes have to be used instead and, not surprisingly, this goes hand in hand with the surge of distressing skin allergies and rashes that so many women, and men, suffer from nowadays.

And I know I am not alone in noticing that many other odours that are man's creation do us no good at all. The fumes that come from industry and traffic can actually cause illness because they continually stress the body. The harmful effects of smog and of lead in petrol are well known. And, unfortunately, we try and camouflage many unpleasant fumes with synthetic flowery commercial sprays, which only make matters worse. I have been told that manufacturers of such 'air fresheners' use in them chemical compounds with anaesthetic properties, such as glyoxal: these deaden the sense of smell for more than an hour, and also irritate the bronchial tubes, which means they can provoke a number of respiratory troubles such as asthma. They also add very potent odoriferous molecules which, because they are so overpowering, drown the unpleasant scent. This gives the impression that it has disappeared although it is actually still there, just temporarily submerged in a sea of other, to my mind, equally noxious smells. No wonder they can make us feel so nauseous.

Other harmful chemicals which are often used in aerosol furniture sprays, window cleansers and so on include chlorine, ammonia and formaldehyde. These also anaesthetise the olfactory organ and, because they are irritant, can cause the appearance of allergies and rashes as severe as bad sunburn.

As the sense of smell is so basic a part of us, I'm sure we all could benefit from a greater awareness of the role it plays in our everyday lives. I would even go so far as to say we ought to re-educate our senses of smell, learning in school, perhaps, how to tell good smells from bad smells, how to differentiate between those that will do us good and those that could possibly harm us. Aromatherapy – literally therapy through aromas – goes a long way towards this re-education.

CHAPTER TWO

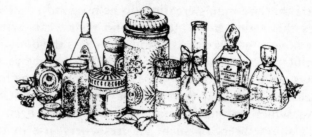

Aromatics in History

If we wish to surround ourselves with pleasant aromas we should turn to nature – to trees, flowers and plants – rather than settling for cheap imitations. Hippocrates is known to have said, 'There is a remedy for every illness to be found in nature,' and I certainly believe he was right and that the plant kingdom, as well as appealing to our sense of smell, is a veritable pharmacopoeia. It not only provides us with the means to heal ourselves, but also demands no rewards for its services.

When an animal is unwell, he will instinctively search for the plants that will heal him. Similarly, primitive man discovered that the plants he ate could affect the way he felt. Although this learning process was slow, the steady growth in his knowledge of how certain plants influenced his system enabled him to cure the illnesses and wounds which afflicted his family and himself. Little wonder therefore that he looked upon plants and flowers with such reverence, believing that each had a soul and that gods resided in the trees. Undoubtedly, too, his sense of smell came into play in his recognition of the different plants, especially those that looked similar, as he began to classify them into those that would heal, cure, kill or provide nourishment.

The first records of such plant classifications are to be

found in the caves of Lascaux in the Dordogne. According to archaeologists' findings the paintings on the cavern walls, made in natural pigments of sepia and ochre, tell of the use of plants as medicines, and date back to about 18000 BC. I was lucky enough to visit these caves during the 1950s, a decade or so after their discovery, when the paintings were still intact, for they have deteriorated thanks to pollution in the air, and have been closed since 1963.

Although we know that plants featured strongly in ancient forms of medicine, it was not until the end of the last century that a French scientist, Professor Gattefossé, actually coined the term 'aromatherapy', by which he meant the therapeutic use of odoriferous substances obtained from flowers, plants and aromatic shrubs, through inhalation and application to the skin. Later Marguerite Maury, a leading authority in the field of aromatherapy, described the aromatic extracts of plants as the 'purest form of living energy that we can insert into man'.

THE ANCIENT EGYPTIANS

We know that aromatic substances played important roles in the medicinal practices of the Hebrew, Greek, Arabic, Chinese and Indian civilisations, but in my opinion aromatherapy was born with the ancient Egyptians. To them, it was a way of life, and we have records dating back to 4500 BC which tell of the use of balsamic substances, perfumed oils, scented barks and resins, spices as well as aromatic vinegars, wines and beers in medicine, liturgy, astrology and embalming.

Translations of the hieroglyphics inscribed on the papyri and steles found in the temple of Edfu indicate that aromatic substances were blended to specific formulations by the high priests and alchemists to make perfumes and medicinal potions. The Papyrus of Ebers shows the wide-

spread use of aromatherapy in pharmacology and path-
ology, for it contains a number of recipes of aromatic mixes
designed to treat a variety of different illnesses. And on the
Papyrus of Edwin Smith, formulations can be found for
restoring youthfulness to ageing men too. We learn that
Egyptian doctors treated hayfever with a mixture of
antimony, aloes, myrrh and honey. Interestingly, the
Egyptians were also surprisingly well versed in the art of
contraception: they would blend together acacia, colo-
quinte, dates and honey, and insert this concoction into the
vagina. There it would ferment to form lactic acid which we
now know acts as a spermicide.

Within the magnificent temples high priests built their
own laboratories where they crushed barks and distilled
flowers to obtain the ingredients for their aromatic potions,
the formulations of which were kept a closely guarded
secret. Seeds like caraway, roots like angelica, barks like
cedarwood, and resins like frankincense were put into wine
or oil, and slowly the aromatic substances would diffuse out
and permeate the liquids which were drunk and burned in
religious ceremonies. The Egyptian priests also used a
sophisticated method of extraction called *enfleurage* by
which the odoriferous molecules are absorbed from the
petals or leaves of plants by grains of sesame seeds. This
technique is still used today in some parts of India.

One of the favourite perfumes was called *kyphi*, a
mixture of sixteen different essences, and this was frequently used in religious ceremonies. Plutarch wrote of it:
'The smell of this perfume penetrates your body by the nose.
It makes you feel well and relaxed, the mind floats and you
find yourself in a dreamy state of happiness, as if listening to
beautiful music.' I would point out that unlike mind-
expanding drugs or alcohol, kyphi allowed the inhaler to
remain alert and responsive, even though he may have felt
as if he had been transported to another plane of con-

sciousness. For this reason the high priests and pharaohs often inhaled it whilst they were meditating, and this practice has been recorded in many inscriptions. Frankincense was also popular and was believed to encourage spiritual awareness, expand the consciousness and develop psychic faculties.

The high priests also acted as spiritual healers capable of treating mental disorders such as depression, mania and acute nervousness, which suggests that their knowledge of how different aromas affect the psyche was incredibly sophisticated.

Illustrations on the temple walls, hieroglyphics engraved on steles and statues all tell of the popularity of the lotus flower in ancient Egypt. It was the sacred flower of Egypt because, in their mythology, it was the first living thing to appear on earth; when the petals unfurled, the supreme god, who represented intellectual rulership, was revealed to them. The lotus grew in abundance along the banks of the Nile, but many other plants and flowers such as the blue orchid, which were highly valued for their aromatic properties, had to be imported from Somalia, Malaysia, India and even as far afield as China. And, because some of the flowers were so highly prized it was usually quite a secretive business.

Such trading flourished under the rule of Queen Hatshepsut (c. 1490–1468 BC), the only woman to become a pharaoh. She adored fine perfumes and encouraged the use of cosmetics and the bold eye make-up that we associate with the ancient Egyptians.

It was not unusual for hundreds of thousands of kilogrammes of plants to be distilled for the creation of scented oils which were then burnt in the temples. On special days the statues of the gods would be covered with scented oils. Each god and goddess had their own fragrance – artemisia for Isis, marrubium for Orus, marjoram for Osiris – and if the pharaohs wished to elicit favours from these supreme beings or thank them for success at war, they would burn these aromatic oils for their pleasure.

When one considers the sheer magnificence of their jewellery, buildings and paintings, it is not difficult to imagine just how sophisticated was the science of aromatherapy in Egyptian times. We learn from translations of hieroglyphics that their vocabulary for the nose was extraordinarily extensive, and the same applied to the many different aromas of plants which were classified into 'notes'. The skilled high priests (or perfumers) would mix together a number of harmonising notes to create a perfume in a manner akin to the composition of a melodious piece of music. Each pharaoh and his family had a number of different perfumes especially composed for them, which were designed to be worn at different times of the day and on special occasions, for they possessed the power to evoke or intensify certain emotions. For example, a perfume for war or battle would stimulate feelings of aggression, whereas another for meditation would promote a state of tranquillity and thoughtfulness.

Different flowers also symbolised different things to the Egyptians, and just as we might send telegrams or cards to one another to wish good health during illness and to show our affection or love, they would send each other the appropriate flower – which to me is a lovely idea.

The embalmer, another important figure in ancient Egypt, was also extremely knowledgeable about the power of plants. He knew that they possessed natural antiseptic and antibiotic properties which could be implemented in the process of preserving human bodies. Each developed his own embalming formulation which he guarded fiercely. Traces of resins like galbanum and spices such as clove, cinnamon and nutmeg have been isolated from the bandages of mummies. Such preservatives were obviously remarkablyeffective. Fragments of intestine examined under the microscope have been found to be completely intact after thousands of years.

The process of embalming is quite fascinating, if rather stomach-turning in places too. It was written about by Herodotus, who discovered that the embalmer would use a fine stick with a hooked end to draw out part of the brain through the nostrils, before injecting a solution of aromatic herbs and solvent into the cavity. He would then open up the abdomen with a sharpened stone from Ethiopia and remove all the viscera which were washed with aromatic palm wine. The abdomen was subsequently filled with myrrh, galbanum and other spices before being stitched up. The viscera went into four different pots called canopic jars, whilst the body was soaked in natron (sodium carbonate solution), left for seventy days, then washed and wrapped in bandages that had been steeped in aromatic resins.

This whole process could take as long as six months before the body was ready to be incarcerated in layer upon layer of elaborately inlaid caskets, before being finally encased in the sarcophagus. Such an elaborate and lengthy treatment was reserved for the high priests and pharaohs, and a much simplified method was employed for those of lowlier origins.

Although the high priests, doctors and embalmers were recognised as being the experts in aromatherapy, even ordinary Egyptians possessed an amazing knowledge of the value of aromatic substances in cooking. They would add spices such as caraway, coriander and aniseed to their breads of millet and barley to make them easier to digest. Mint, marjoram and parsley were also widely used. Often they would substitute onions for meat – a bulb was invariably found beside the tomb of a mummy. Garlic was also valued for its bactericidal properties to stave off the ever-present threat of epidemic. A translation of an inscription on the Pyramid of Cheops, 4500 BC, states that every morning each slave would be given a clove of garlic by his master to provide him with the strength and good health needed for its construction.

AROMATICS TODAY

Even today, although most of us do not think about it, we practise aromatherapy in everyday life. We take flowers or a plant to a friend who is ill; we sit next to a rose garden or under a linden tree when we want to relax, for unconsciously we are aware that their fragrances have a soothing effect on our nerves.

When we cook, we use root ginger or rosemary, although perhaps we do not realise that the aromas they produce trigger the secretion of gastric juices which in turn facilitates good digestion. In addition, the essential oils that are released from herbs during cooking also make meat more digestible and their antibacterial properties will counteract any toxins that may be present.

If we have flu or a cold we rub eucalyptus in an oily base onto the chest, for its vapours help to clear the head, and a sugary cinnamon drink will always ease a cough or sore throat. And, when we want to pamper ourselves we add scented essences to the bath, knowing that this will help us unwind at the end of a hectic day.

CHAPTER THREE

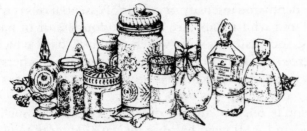

Essential Oils

The odoriferous substances which are found in wild or cultivated plants are called essential oils. These are frequently referred to as the 'soul' of the plant or as its hormones, but they could also be likened to the pheromones that are secreted by humans. If you take a few leaves of lavender or rosemary and rub or squeeze them between your fingers, you will smell the distinctive aroma of the essential oils that have oozed out of them onto your skin.

Most flowers, seeds, barks, grains, roots and resins as well as leaves contain essential oils, usually in rather minute quantities. Sometimes several essential oils can be extracted from the same plant. The orange tree, for instance, contains one essential oil called orange in the rind or skin of the fruit; another called petitgrain is obtained from the leaves, and yet another known as neroli is responsible for the wonderful scent of the flowers. Each oil has a different smell and different therapeutic properties.

Often it is the smallest flowers which are the most intensely perfumed. At the beginning of this century it was thought that if plants were bred to produce larger flowers, they would have a stronger fragrance than the original smaller ones. However, because the plant uses more energy to grow the larger blooms, it actually produces fewer essential oils, so such experiments failed miserably.

The depth and intensity of colour of essential oils is quite varied and whilst some are almost colourless or of pastel shades, such as camomile, which is bluish, basil which is light green and Bulgarian rose which is pale pink, others are deeply pigmented: patchouli is brown, violet leaves are very dark green, and rose is orange-red.

Essential oils are unlike other vegetable oils such as almond and sunflower, because they are lighter than water (with the exception of garlic and cinnamon), and are usually highly fluid (although some are more viscous, of a honey-like consistency). The odoriferous molecules tend to be extremely volatile because of their unusually high number of free electrons, so they evaporate quickly, especially when warmed. A test you can try for yourself involves simply applying a few drops of essential oil of lavender to a piece of ordinary white writing paper. The patch will be slightly coloured and you will see it disappear in a very short time as the aromatic substances vaporise and disperse to scent the air.

EXTRACTING THE ESSENTIAL OILS

Essential oils can be obtained from plants in a number of ways, and the right method is important for it will influence the ultimate quality and theraupeutic properties of the oils.

Maceration

An example of this technique is *enfleurage*, often used for flowers like jasmine and tuberose. High quality flowers or petals that have not been damaged in any way are spread out on a tray lined with fat or vegetable oil. The flowers are left for sixteen to seventy-two hours, then replaced by fresh ones at regular intervals, until the fat is saturated with their perfume. This is a painstaking process that can last for up to three months before the aromatic substances can be separated – in a process called *défleurage* – from the fat with a solvent and purified. Essential oils extracted in this way tend to be of a superior quality to those obtained by distillation and, consequently, they are usually more expensive.

Distillation

Distillation has been used as a method of extracting essential oils from plant material for thousands of years. The ancient Egyptians were known to place their raw material and some water in a large clay pot. Heat was applied and the steam that formed had to pass through layers of cotton or linen cloth placed in the neck before escaping. The essential oils became trapped in this material, and all that had to be done to obtain them was to squeeze out the cloth periodically. It is still the most common means of extraction: steam is passed over the leaves or flowers, possibly in a vacuum or under pressure, so that the essential oils within them vaporise. When the steam is cooled, the essential oils condense and, because they are not water soluble, they separate and can be collected quite easily.

Dissolving

Sometimes it is preferable to use a volatile solvent such as alcohol for extracting gums and resins like galbanum and myrrh. In the case of fresh flowers and plants, however, ether or benzine may be used instead.

Pressing

This technique is not commonly employed commercially, but it can be used to squeeze the essential oils from the rinds and peels of fruits like oranges and lemons.

FROM FLOWER TO ESSENTIAL OIL

If I trace the pathway from lavender flowers to pure essential oil, you will see why it is far superior in quality and also more expensive than any artificial copy.

Lavender is a member of the labiate family which, together with plants falling into the categories of umbelliferous, myrtaceae, rutaceous, lauriferous, terebinthos and coniferous, is particularly rich in essential oils. The essential oil should be highly scented and very pleasant, varying in colour from dark yellow to dark greeny yellow. Its principal constituents are esters such as linalyl and geranyle, alcohols like garaniol, linalol and borneol, as well as terpenes like limonene and binene (see following for composition of essential oils).

It takes approximately 200 kg (440 lb) of fresh flowers to obtain 1 kg (just over 2 lb) of essential oil, and because the flowers do not travel very well, extraction often has to take place on the spot, soon after the flowers have been gathered.

The quality of the oil depends on a number of different interacting factors. The *time* of picking is vital, and once the flowers are ready, harvesting should be completed in a matter of two weeks, for if there is delay the odoriferous substances will be lost. Also, like wine, the quality of essential oils varies from year to year, so there are good, and not so good, 'vintages'. This is not really surprising when you consider that the climate, the composition of the soil, geographic location – the altitude, whether the lavender is grown in a secluded valley, or on an exposed mountain slope – all play a role in influencing the ultimate quality of the essential oil. For example, flowers picked from plants living in a natural environment, as they do in parts of Persia or 750–1,500 metres up in the Alps of southern France, give a more subtle perfume than their cultivated English counterparts. This is because the French lavender is richer in linolyle acetate, which gives rise to a fruitier and sweeter note, considered pleasanter than the camphoric English lavender with its higher proportion of lineol – and it is, as a result, much more expensive.

Sometimes the colour, as well as the smell, of the oil can make it easy to tell a good from a poor quality one, the best being a dark or greeny yellow shade. Paler and more insipid-smelling oils are not so desirable, so other constituents are sometimes added to alter them which, of course, has the adverse effect of diminishing their therapeutic properties.

THE COMPOSITION OF ESSENTIAL OILS

Each essential oil is made up of numerous different organic molecules which dissolve in alcohols, oils, emulsifiers, ether or chloroform. The individual aroma and therapeutic properties of each essential oil depends on the combination and concentration of these constituent molecules, which belong to several different chemical families.

Alcohols

Menthol in mint; linalol in ylang ylang and lavender; geraniol in geranium and rose; nerol in neroli and orange; borneol in lavender and pine.

Aldehydes

Citral in lemongrass and mandarin; benzoic in benzoin and laurel; citronellal in lemon, eucalyptus and melissa; vanilline in vanilla and styrax.

Acids

Cinnamic acid in styrax; benzoic acid in ylang ylang.

Phenols

Eugenol in clove; safrol in sassafras; thymol in thyme; gaicol in gaiac.

Esters

Benzyl acetate in styrax; linalyl in bergamot and lavender.

Acetones

Cineol in eucalyptus; jasmone in neroli and jasmine; irone in iris.

Terpenes

Pinene in cypress; camphene in petitgrain and juniper; terpineol in coriander and elemi; phellandrene in lemon and sage; limonene in lemon, carro and mint.

Each essential oil is an incredibly complex substance for it contains a number of different alcohols, esters, phenols and so on. Eucalyptus, for example, is made up of 250 different constituents, which is why it is almost impossible to reproduce it exactly with synthetic ingredients. The therapeutic value of an essential oil also depends largely on the synergistic reaction between the component molecules, which is why man-made imitations never have the same power to heal as their natural counterparts.

THE PROPERTIES OF ESSENTIAL OILS

All essential oils, whether they come from flowers, fruits, resins or barks, have antibiotic, antiseptic, anti-inflammatory and anti-viral properties to a greater or lesser degree.

The ancient Egyptians used essential oils in embalming because they knew of their ability to prevent the proliferation of the microbes which cause flesh to decompose. Hippocrates, too, was aware of their antibacterial properties, for when an epidemic of plague broke out in Athens, he urged the townspeople to burn aromatic plants at the corners of the streets to protect themselves and to prevent the plague from spreading.

Centuries later, when the plague reared its ugly head in England (in 1665–6), Charles II's doctor also declared that every householder should fumigate his rooms with aromatic essences to fight this scourge. At this time, it was common practice to wear pomanders containing garlic and cloves around the neck, to give protection.

Even up until the last war essential oils of clove, lemon, thyme and camomile were employed as natural disinfectants and antiseptics to fumigate maternity wards of hospitals and sterilise instruments used in surgery and dentistry.

When Sir Alexander Fleming discovered the antibiotic penicillin in 1928, it too was 'natural', isolated from a culture of mould (etymologically, antibiotic means 'against life', thus the ability to destroy bacteria). Today, of course, natural penicillin is no longer used, for long ago its constituents were identified and it is now synthesised in the laboratory. Perhaps this is the reason why so many people have allergic reactions to penicillin resulting in eczema and swelling: the artificial variety is considerably stronger than its natural counterpart.

Although the naturally derived antibiotics like essential oils act slowly, they do not only kill the bacteria or virus, but also stimulate the body's immune system to strengthen resistance to further attack. Taking strong drugs, on the other hand, is rather like cracking a nut with a sledgehammer, for they not only kill the harmful bacteria, they also destroy the beneficial ones present in our intestines. These are responsible for maintaining a good environment for digestion to take place and for making significant quantities of B complex vitamins.

The trouble is that, nowadays, we have come to expect instant cures and think that the only antibiotics of any value are made synthetically and come in pill form. Thus many find it hard to believe that the essential oils from plants are actually just as effective, if not more so. They may take longer to show results, but as it may have taken a long time for the symptoms of the illness to reveal themselves, so they are unlikely to disappear overnight. There *are no* miracle cures.

Scientists working in a number of different fields around the world – doctors, professors of medicine, chemists and biologists – have carried out laboratory tests which increasingly prove – and confirm – that essential oils have the ability to prevent the proliferation of harmful bacteria. Such tests involve adding a few drops of essential oil, such as lavender, to a culture of microbes. The time it takes to destroy the colony of bacilli gives a good indication of how strongly antiseptic or antibiotic that particular essential oil is.

It is certain constituent molecules that lend an essential oil its antibacterial properties, and they vary in efficacy. Phenol, for example, is the strongest, and because it makes up 80 per cent of Spanish oregano this essential oil is consequently a powerful antibiotic and antiseptic, as are eucalyptus, clove, niaouli, thyme, sandalwood, lemon, cinnamon, lavender and mint. Then come the aldehydes, alcohols, esters and finally the acids, in order of diminishing potency. I should point out, however, that the natural essential oil is infinitely superior to pure phenol because, as I mentioned earlier, the presence of the other molecules in the oil reinforces its action.

Luckily, we do not have epidemics of plague to cope with as they did in the past, but we do still suffer from frequent colds and flu, especially during the winter months, which can be extremely debilitating, and essential oils can be tremendously helpful for keeping such ills at bay, and for treating the symptoms too.

Another useful property of essential oils is their ability to soothe inflammation and reduce swelling. The Egyptians knew of this property too, classifying essential oils from plants according to their colour tones and heat, as opposed to their constituent molecules. To them they were either hot or cold, dark or clear, damp or dry, and heavy or light. As in the philosophy of Chinese medicine, which divides all things into yin and yang, they believed that balance was absolutely crucial to the harmonious functioning of the body and mind. So, for an affliction such as rheumatism, or a swelling caused by water retention, a hot and dry oil such as rosemary or ginger would be applied to redress the balance. When put into practice, this theory still does work exceptionally well.

The following is a selection of the more common essential oils and their properties.

Benzoin

This essence has a lovely scent reminiscent of vanilla and is often used as a fixative in perfume. It is extracted from the resin of trees, native to Malaysia, Java and Borneo, that grow to about 20 metres (60 feet) in height, each tree yielding 500–600 g (about 1–1¼ lb) of resin. It is useful for treating respiratory problems such as asthma, when breathing in is difficult, and skin problems such as melanosis when skin becomes pigmented.

For inhalation, add a few drops of benzoin to 500 ml (a scant pint) of water. For a massage oil, add 1 drop to 2 teaspoons of an oil such as almond.

Bergamot

Bergamot belongs to the orange tree family and was discovered by Christopher Columbus when he went to the Canary Islands. Bergamot now grows further afield as well, in southern Italy, Sicily, and along the Ivory Coast of Africa. The essential oil, distilled from the peel of the fruit, has a lovely emerald-green colour, and a spicy lemon scent. It has strong antiseptic, tonic and stomachic properties (good for fighting infections, for boosting the whole body, and for the stomach).

Care should be taken when applying it externally, however, because one of its constituent molecules, furocoumarine, can provoke abnormal pigmentation of the skin when exposed to the sun.

Cajput

The name and oil derive from the Malay *kayu-puti*, white tree, which grows abundantly in Malaysia and the Molucca Islands. The essential oils are extracted from the leaves and buds, and have a very aromatic, hot smell. Cajput is a strong antiseptic and benefits the pulmonary, intestinal and urinary tracts.

For treating cystitis, add 3 drops to a bath, or massage with an oil made by adding 3 drops of cajput to 4–5 teaspoons of soya oil. In inhalations it helps treat colds. Add 3–4 drops to 500 ml (a scant pint) of warm water. Add 2 drops to 2 teaspoons of oil for a massage oil to give relief from rheumatic conditions.

Camomile

The essential oils, distilled from freshly dried camomile flowers, have a lovely blue colour which later turns greenish yellow. Camomile was a sacred flower in Egypt and was offered to please the sun god, Ra, and used as a remedy for fever.

It is a good tonic, digestive, sedative (reduces and calms a fever) and antiseptic, and promotes the cicatrisation of wounds thanks to one of its constituents, azulene. Camomile helps to treat skin troubles by soothing the inflammation of eczema, and acne conditions. It is also good for stings and bites, cystitis, amenorrhoea, dysmenorrhoea, bronchitis, asthma, coughs, migraine and the neuralgia of flu.

For external use on the face, add 2 drops to 2 teaspoons of soya oil. For a body massage oil, mix 2 drops of camomile with 2 drops of rosemary in 4–5 teaspoons of soya oil. This can help to relieve rheumatic aches and pains. As a tonic and stimulant for children and old people who have been ill, add 5–6 drops to a warm bath.

Cardamom

The essential oils come from the distillation of the seeds found in the fruits of various plants belonging to the ginger family. They have a lovely fresh smell which neutralises the odour of garlic. Dr Leclerc, a famous French naturopath and herbalist, believed that cardamom was one of the best carminatives (an aid for wind and flatulence), digestives, stimulants, nerve and heart tonics.

It is also an effective diuretic and is even better when used with other essences such as juniper which reinforces its action. When chewed, cardamom seeds provide an excellent remedy for halitosis.

Cedarwood

The cedarwood tree comes from North Africa, Morocco and Algeria, and its wood has a lovely fragrance. The essential oil has a syrupy consistency and, like sandalwood, is balsamic. The ancient Egyptians used it frequently in embalming.

It is antiseptic and benefits the urinary system, providing a remedy for cystitis and bladder infections. It is also good for the respiratory system and treats bronchitis. Cedarwood can help skin troubles like eczema, and could be used in hair care to treat alopecia. It is a general tonic and possesses aphrodisiac properties as well.

For the bath, use 5–7 drops of essence. For inhalation, use a few drops in about 500 ml (a scant pint) of hot water. For a massage oil for the scalp and face add 2–4 drops of essence to 2 teaspoons of oil. You could also add a few drops to your shampoo if you have problems with falling hair.

Cypress

Cypress trees come from the East and all the Mediterranean countries. The essences, which are obtained by distillation of the leaves, twigs and cones of the tree, are slightly yellow and their perfume is agreeable and tenacious. In ancient Egypt cypress essential oils were valued for their medicinal properties, and the wood itself was used to make the sarcophagi.

The essences help to treat circulatory problems such as varicose veins and haemorrhoids, and they also benefit the urinary system. Add 4–6 drops of essence to a warm bath or foot bath. For bad circulation massage the legs every day with 2–4 drops of cypress in 2 teaspoons of soya oil.

Eucalyptus

The eucalyptus tree originated in Australia and was later introduced to North Africa and the Mediterranean coastline. The essential oils extracted from its silvery leaves are pale yellow in colour, have a fresh, aromatic smell, and are highly medicinal. The essence's principal constituent is eucalyptol which gives it strong antiseptic properties.

It is excellent for respiratory problems, providing an effective remedy for coughs, asthma, bronchitis, catarrhal discharge, and the fever which accompanies flu. It can be used to treat cystitis, skin problems, and to heal cuts and burns. It also acts as a stimulant for the nervous system.

For asthma, flu, bronchial and rheumatic problems inhale 2 drops of eucalyptus mixed with 1 drop of niaouli and 1 drop of pine – or add 5–10 drops to a bath for rheumatics. For skin problems mix 2 drops in 2 teaspoons of soya oil, and rub vigorously into any affected area. For a natural fumigant when someone is ill at home, boil some eucalyptus leaves in water, and let the vapours disperse through the house. Similarly, especially for bronchitics, leave an infusion of leaves (or of the oil) near the bed at night.

Frankincense

This essential oil is extracted from the gum resin obtained by making an incision in a tree which grows in Arabia and south-east Africa. The essential oil is yellowish in colour and has a balsamic aroma. Its perfume becomes slightly lemony when mixed with myrrh and aromatic spices, and the sweet-smelling smoke exuded when this mixture is burned was often used in religious ceremonies. It is a good nerve tonic, antiseptic, and pectoral (good for the chest).

Add 5–6 drops to a bath, or place a few drops on a glass slide left by the radiator, if you want to relax or meditate.

Galbanum

The essence comes from a gum resin obtained from a species of fennel which grows in Persia. It is yellow in colour, and has a lovely hot, pungent, aromatic fragrance.

It can be used to treat skin problems such as abscesses and inflammation, and also encourages the formation of scar tissue. For an oil to rub into affected areas, mix a few drops in a peach kernel or almond oil.

Geranium

Geranium originates from Africa and in 1690 was brought to Europe. The essence, often called geranium Bourbon-la Réunion (from the island near Madagascar), is usually colourless but can be yellowish green, and has a strong but agreeable smell. An imitation of its aroma is frequently made by mixing a few of its constituent molecules with essences of sandalwood and citronella.

Geranium essence is good for skin problems such as frostbite, dermatitis and inflammation. It helps the cicatrisation of wounds and treats haemorrhoids and bad circulation.

For a skin massage oil, mix 2–3 drops in 2 teaspoons of soya oil. For haemorrhoids apply 1 drop mixed with cold cream. For inflammation of the breast when breast-feeding, mix 3 drops into some cold cream.

Lavender

Lavender originated from Persia, the Canary Islands and the Mediterranean coast, and many different varieties grow throughout Europe today.

Lavender essence is effective in the treatment of skin troubles such as bruises, frostbite, erythema, acne and dermatitis, and also reduces swelling. It brings relief to rheumatic conditions, and is particularly good when mixed with juniper, cypress or ginger. Add 2 drops of each to 2–3 teaspoons of soya oil and massage into the affected area. For skin conditions, add 3 drops to 2 teaspoons of oil.

It was Dr Gattefossé, one of the founding fathers of aromatherapy, who discovered the marvellous burn-healing powers of lavender. When he severely burned his hand in the laboratory, he plunged it, accidentally, into the nearest bowl – full of essential oil of lavender. The pain ceased and the burn healed very quickly thereafter.

For bad burns, apply pure essence of lavender straight-away, wrap the affected part in gauze or muslin (to let the skin breathe), and repeat two to three times per day, about every four hours. For less severe burns, when cooking for instance, dab on lavender oil immediately, and cover. If you have no essential oil available, get some lavender flowers or leaves from the garden, apply to the burn, and wrap as above.

Lemongrass

This sweet-scented grass is cultivated in India, the African Congo, the Seychelles, Indonesia, Sri Lanka and Brazil, principally for seasoning food. The essential oil has a lemony aroma and its main constituents are citral (strongly antiseptic) and geraniol.

It helps treat any infections accompanied by a temperature, it gives relief from migraine headaches, and benefits anyone with excessively perspiring feet or athlete's foot.

For a foot bath, add a few drops of lemongrass to a bowl of water, then rub into the feet an oil made by adding 3 drops of essence to 1 teaspoon of soya oil.

Always use lemongrass as a home antiseptic instead of the chemical varieties, but only externally.

Melissa

This plant is cultivated throughout Europe and grows wild in woods and fields. The essence is more or less colourless, but can have a slight yellow hue, and smells lemony.

It is anti-spasmodic, stimulant (for the nervous system), and tonic for the cardiac system or heart. It helps treat depression, nervous anxiety and palpitations as well as neuralgia and sciatica, so it is particularly beneficial to many elderly people.

Rub into the chest an oil made by adding 5 drops of essence to 2 teaspoons soya oil. This can be used as a general body oil too. Add 6 drops to the bath for nerves, anxiety or palpitations. When depressed, drink an infusion of the plant. Add 2 pinches of the plant to 500 ml (a scant pint) of boiling water. Let stand for 10 minutes, and sweeten with honey if liked.

Myrrh

Essence of myrrh comes from a yellowy brown gum resin and originates from Arabia and Persia. The essence itself may be any shade of yellow, from very pale through to a deep golden colour, and it has a highly aromatic and camphor-like smell. Myrrh has been used in religious ceremonies since antiquity, and the ancient Egyptians, who called it '*phun*', used it for embalming purposes as well.

Its principal constituents are terpenes, pinenes, phenols, etc.; it has good antiseptic properties, reduces inflammation, and treats skin problems such as acne and dermatitis. For external application, make an oil by adding 2–4 drops of essence to 2 teaspoons of soya oil.

Neroli

Essence of neroli is obtained by distilling the fresh flowers of the bitter orange tree. The most esteemed oil comes from the bitter orange, *citrus bigaradia*, and is known as neroli bigarade, whilst another, called neroli portugal, comes from a sweet orange tree. Neroli is a very expensive essential oil (1 ton of flowers is needed to produce 1 kg or 2 lb of oil), and it has a yellowish colour which can turn brown when exposed to light. It is rich in alcohols like nerol, linalol and geraniol.

Neroli is highly beneficial to the nervous system, and effectively treats anxiety and nervous depression. Because it has a slightly hypnotic effect, it induces sleep and acts as a natural tranquilliser. Add 4 drops to a bath before going to bed, and for a sleep-inducing drink, a few drops can be added to orange-blossom tea sweetened with honey. If depressed and anxious – or simply leading too hectic a lifestyle! – massage into the skin an oil made by adding 4–6 drops of essence to 2 teaspoons of soya oil.

Neroli is also a natural blood cleanser – taken as an infusion of the flowers – and helps improve bad circulation, when the above oil should be massaged in every day. A few drops of neroli added to baths for a week prior to menstruation can help alleviate the symptoms of pre-menstrual tension.

Patchouli

Essence of patchouli comes from the dried branches of a plant which originated in Malaysia and the Seychelles. The essential oil is brown and viscous, and has a strong, persistent smell. It is often used as a fixative in perfumes. It is a good antiseptic and can be applied wherever there is infection. It reduces inflammation, soothes burns, and helps to treat skin problems such as seborrhoea, acne, dermatitis and allergic reactions.

For the skin, make an oil by adding 2 drops of essence to 2 teaspoons of almond oil. Add a few drops to your shampoo if you have excessively oily hair.

Pine

The essential oils come from both the resins and needles of the pine tree, of which there are 150 varieties. I consider the best essences are those extracted from the needles of pines that grow in Scandinavia and Russia. The essence is very pale yellow and has a lovely balsamic smell which it owes to its principal constituents – pinene, sylvestrene, phellandrene and cadinene.

Pine is an excellent antiseptic which benefits the respiratory system (helping flu, colds and bronchitis), and the urinary tract (helping treat cystitis). It has a revitalising action and benefits children and adults alike.

It is also anti-rheumatic and particularly effective when mixed with lemon or juniper. Add 2 drops of each to 2 teaspoons of soya oil, and rub into the affected area.

For inhalation to ease the symptoms of flu and colds, add 2 drops of pine, 2 drops of niaouli and 2 drops of eucalyptus to 500 ml (a scant pint) of hot water.

Rose

The rose initially came from the East, but now there are

many hundreds of different varieties which grow nearly everywhere. However, only three reproduce faithfully to give true perfume of rose, and they are rose centifolia, rose damask and rose gallica. Throughout history rose has been the perfume of kings and pharoahs. It was also used both as an aphrodisiac for women and, ironically, in religious ceremonies.

It usually takes about 2 tons of rose petals to produce just 1 kg (2 lb) of essential oil, and for this reason it is one of the most expensive of the essences. The best essences to look for are Bulgarian, Moroccan, Oriental rose and rose de Grasse. It is not surprising that imitations of rose are often made by mixing some of its constituent molecules with essential oils of lemongrass, geranium and citronella.

Rose is a general tonic and fortifier, and has a particularly effective action on the nervous, circulatory and respiratory systems. It is good for all skin problems, from eczema, wrinkles and dryness, to puffiness and congestion of the pores. For skin problems mix 2–3 drops in 2 teaspoons of almond oil.

It is also believed to be a sexual stimulant for women, and may help those who complain of frigidity. Make a body oil for special occasions by adding 3–6 drops to 3–4 teaspoons of soya oil.

Sassafras

This small tree or bush belonging to the laurel family grows in North America. The essential oils are usually obtained from its bark and roots, although they can also be distilled from the flowers and leaves. The oils are reddish-yellow in colour and smell strongly of safrol, which is pungent and aromatic with a hint of fennel and anise. It was considered sacred by the American Iroquois Indians, who used it for its medicinal properties.

Sassafras is a tonic combating fatigue and nervous depression, and is beneficial when used after strenuous exercise. It also possesses diuretic and anti-rheumatic properties, and helps treat lumbago and back problems. Make a massage oil by adding 2–4 drops to 2 teaspoons of oil, or add 4–6 drops to a bath.

NB   This essence should not be used by pregnant women.

Ylang Ylang

These trees – known as perfume trees – are native to the Far East, the Philippines and Malaysia, but are also found in Asia, the Seychelles, Tahiti and India. The essential oil, which is distilled from the fresh flowers, is pale yellow and has an exquisite perfume. In the past the flowers were mixed in coconut oil and used to improve the condition of the hair, to soothe insect bites, and to fight infections. The pure essences were also used to treat malaria. Ylang ylang is antiseptic, aphrodisiac and tonic to the nervous system.

Add 4–6 drops to a bath, or 4 drops to 2 teaspoons of soya oil, and perfume your body with it for special occasions. Also add 3–4 drops to 60 ml (about 2 fl. oz) of gentle shampoo.

CHAPTER FOUR

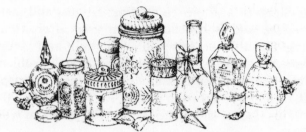

Aromatherapy and Illness

Aromatherapy is the therapeutic use of odoriferous substances obtained from flowers, plants and aromatic shrubs.
Not only can it be used to treat and cure illness effectively
but, perhaps even more importantly, it can also help to
prevent us from losing our good health in the first place.

Today we fight a constant battle to stay well. Many of us
live and work in large cities or towns where we are, in a
sense, trapped in confined spaces which constrict our
freedom of movement and diminish the exercise we should
be getting to keep us fit. Cars, automatic washing machines,
desk jobs, all encourage this sedentary existence. We are
under constant bombardment from radiation, which has a
damaging effect on the chemistry of all the cells in our
bodies. Even the television which we spend so much time
watching emits a significant degree of radioactive waves.

Nowadays people experience a good deal of psychological stress which comes from the anxiety of a demanding
job, and the even greater fear that that job might be lost.
More and more women pursue careers, often on top of
running a home and looking after a family, which puts
demands on them that were unknown even fifty years ago.

In addition, there is the ever-escalating quantity of traffic
with its noise and pollution. All these things act as stressors
which diminish the energy reserves needed to fight off illness

and stay healthy. Of course, it is impossible to turn back the clock, and it would be foolish to refuse to accept these technological advances. Instead, we have to adapt ourselves to cope with the ever-changing environment, and this is where aromatherapy is so helpful. For by inhaling the essences, massaging plant oils into the skin and taking them internally, the natural resistance to stress and illness can be built up.

In a way, aromatherapy is giving back the environment which we miss by living in towns and cities, as it recreates the fragrances of the trees and flowers which would naturally surround us in the country. I believe that plants are living beings, each possessing its own energy potential which, according to the laws of nature, may be transmitted to us. This is one of the reasons why they offer the perfect remedy for treating and curing our ills.

We are more aware today than ever before of the potential side-effects of some drugs, especially the anti-depressant and tranquillising pills that are frequently resorted to when pressures of job or life in general become too great to bear. Anyone reluctant to turn to tranquillisers, antibiotics or other pills to help them alleviate seemingly minor problems as diverse as nervousness, insomnia, headaches, influenza and swollen joints, will find aroma-therapy invaluable. It provides the means to treat such ailments before they turn into much more serious kinds of illness. It is also an ideal means of curing young children's ills and injuries, and a daily application of plant oils will even help alleviate the pains of rheumatism and arthritis from which so many older people suffer.

THE ODOUR OF ILLNESS

To me it is a fascinating fact that, not only does your sense of smell diminish when you are ill, but your body smell alters as well. Research in the field of endocrinology has revealed that different diseases have their own brands of smell which are, not surprisingly, in general rather noxious. For instance, scurvy smells of decaying meat, smallpox of putrescence, eczema and impetigo of rotting skin. People with diphtheria have a sweet and rather nauseous odour, and typhoid sufferers have a surprisingly pleasant aroma reminiscent of fresh bread. Cancer is also believed to change your body smell for the worse, and it is said that when Freud suffered from cancer of the throat, his favourite dog was unable to stand his smell and would not go near him.

The body has a large number of different secretions and excretions in the form of sweat, sebum, mucus, vaginal secretions, faeces and urine. The odour of these (due to pheromones present in them) determines the aroma of skin, hair and clothes, and can be subtly influenced by mood, diet, the amount of exercise taken and, in women, by their monthly cycle. But when one or more of these bodily secretions takes on an unfamiliar, unpleasant aroma, it is a good indication of some kind of glandular imbalance or organ dysfunction and should be heeded. It is also interesting to know that when drugs, medicinal or otherwise, are taken that they too can affect the quality of body smells.

Halitosis, or bad breath, is one of the first signs of something amiss. It can mean liver trouble, inadequate digestion of food, tooth decay, respiratory problems, gum infections, inflammation of the throat, catarrhal discharge, or sinus trouble. So apart from being rather anti-social, it is also a sort of early-warning system, and action should be taken before the problem gets out of hand.

Smelly feet can be caused by the presence of undesirable bacteria and fungi – such as the kind responsible for athlete's foot – but can also indicate an emotional problem: profuse sweating often goes hand in hand with worry, fear or anxiety. A good way of combating this problem is to bathe the feet in a mixture of witch-hazel and pine.

Many people have a problem with flatulence, which can be particularly embarrassing, and at times very anti-social. We all swallow a certain amount of oxygen and nitrogen from the air which has to be dispelled, and this is perfectly natural. In times of stress, however, we are likely to take in more air because we speak faster and gasp, which is why we are sometimes more gaseous when anxious, but again this is not unusual.

However, other gases can be formed in the intestines by the fermentation of certain foods and they are of a particularly distasteful nature because of their sulphurous notes. This variety spells trouble with the digestive processes. Some people do not possess the enzymes which digest the sugar (lactose) in milk and as a result a good deal of stomach discomfort such as bloating and flatulence occurs because of the gas produced through fermentation. These people have an inherent intolerance to dairy produce and would be better off avoiding it completely. Gluten can also spell trouble for some people, who are unable to digest it properly – known as coeliac disease, and usually diagnosed in infancy – and they should avoid wheat products and, to a lesser extent, other grains such as barley, oats, and rye.

Many other foods can also encourage flatulence, but this is perfectly normal. Take beans, for instance. Scientists interested in the phenomenon found that people who lived primarily on a diet of beans for seven days produced exceedingly large quantities of wind – which no doubt accounts for the bad reputation they have acquired! This is because the sugar they contain tends to ferment in the intestine. Action can be taken to prevent this by cooking them with aromatic herbs, which aid their digestion. The same applies to certain other vegetables such as cabbage,

Brussels sprouts, cauliflower, broccoli, turnips, cucumber, radish and onions, but once again, if cooked and seasoned properly, this disconcerting phenomenon can be avoided. Changes also occur in the vaginal secretions, which are more copious at certain times of the month than at others, and this is perfectly normal. However, a white or yellow discharge which smells rather disagreeable indicates something is not right, for it can be formed as a consequence of vaginal irritation caused by the presence of bacteria or fungi such as *trichomonas vaginalis, hemophillius vaginalis,* and *candida albicans.* Interestingly, women who take the pill seem to be more susceptible to this affliction because the hormones contained in the pill alter the pH of the vaginal secretions, making them more alkaline, thus providing the perfect breeding ground for such bacteria. Antibiotic medications will encourage this problem as well, as they kill the protective bacteria which keep the harmful ones at bay, thus making the vaginal secretions more alkaline.

So the pill and antibiotics are not a good combination. Women suffering from vaginal irritation should be aware of this and can help themselves, not only with essential oils (see Chapter Six), but also by avoiding wearing nylon next to their skin, or tight jeans: both prevent the skin from breathing properly, creating a good environment within which these bacteria can thrive.

HOW TO USE ESSENTIAL OILS

Essential oils can be applied in several different ways to prevent illness, and to treat the symptoms that accompany various ailments. They can be massaged into the skin, added to a warm bath, inhaled as a vapour, or taken internally, for all these methods will help them to reach the inner parts of the body which need to be protected or healed. The olfactory organ and the sense of smell are vital factors, of course, but the prime aid to good and effective use of essential oils is the skin.

Few people realise that the skin is the largest organ of the body; in a person weighing around 75 kg (165 lb), the skin will constitute approximately 3 kg (6½ lb) of this weight, whereas the liver is responsible for a mere 1.5 kg (just over 3 lb). On the whole, the skin is only about 1–2 mm deep (about the thickness of a 1p coin) but on the palms of the hands and soles of the feet it is greater, and can even be as thick as 4 mm at the top of the neck, near the skull.

Skin is composed of two distinct layers: the outer epidermis, the only part we see, which is continually renewing itself as new cells are formed and old ones are shed from the surface; and a deeper layer called the dermis which contains the connective tissue that lends skin its remarkable strength, suppleness and pliancy. The skin is endowed with a very good supply of blood which is brought to the surface by tiny capillaries, and is also teeming with nerve endings which are responsible for our perception of touch and pain.

One of the skin's main functions is the elimination of wastes, of sweat, and of excess sebum, the lubricating oil produced by the sebaceous glands (which are most active during puberty, causing greasy skin and spots). These are excreted through tiny pores which cover the entire surface of the skin. Oxygen and carbon dioxide also pass in and out of the skin, in a kind of respiration akin to that which takes place in the lungs.

Exactly how essential oils are taken up by the skin still remains rather a mystery, but it is quite possible that they pass in through the pores which produce sweat and sebum. And because the odoriferous molecules of an essential oil are extremely volatile, it is possible that they diffuse through the skin in the same way as other gases.

Many are sceptical of the ability of the skin to absorb essential oils, or any other substances for that matter, seeing it as an impenetrable barrier. But this is not the case: essential oils have the ability to penetrate right into the deep layers of the skin and from there travel to the various organs, glands and tissues of the body. Once they have passed through the epidermis, they seep into the small capillaries in the dermis and are carried all around the body in the blood. They are also taken up by the lymph fluid which bathes every cell in the body. Experiments with guinea pigs have shown that if a few drops of lavender oil labelled with a radioactive substance are applied to a patch of shaved skin, when the animal is killed and dissected about an hour and a half later, the essential oil can be detected in the kidneys. A simple test you can carry out yourself which shows just how effectively essential oils are absorbed and transported around the body, is to rub the soles of your feet (or those of a friend) with a clove of garlic. A few hours later you will be able to smell garlic on the breath.

Different essential oils are picked up and fixed in different parts of the body. Violet leaves, for example, are found concentrated in the kidneys, rosemary in the intestines, and sandalwood in the bladder, whilst neroli and ylang ylang, known for their soothing and relaxing properties, are attracted to the nervous system. It seems that certain organs or glands which are in need of help selectively take up different essential oils and use them in the same way as they would utilise the vitamins and minerals they need to function properly. This is perhaps the reason why essential oils have gained a reputation for being able to boost a sluggish organ into action.

Because it is in continual contact with the external environment, the skin also plays an essential role in forming a first line of defence against the bacteria and viruses in the air around us. Deep beneath the skin there are many protective bacteria, and these find their way into the dermis.

Their job is to keep the harmful bacteria such as coli bacteria, staphylococci and streptococci, which land on the surface of the epidermis, at bay. Washing the skin with a mild soap and water helps to flush away these harmful bacteria, together with the excess sebum and sweat that accumulate on the surface of the skin. However, washing with too strong a detergent can also destroy the good bacteria: strong peeling treatments, ultraviolet light and skin trauma such as burns also reduce the number of good bacteria and leave the skin open to attack by the harmful ones.

Thanks to their natural antibacterial and anti-viral properties, daily application of essential oils can build up the skin's natural resistance to the illnesses such germs can bring. When they are applied to the skin, they should first be diluted in a vegetable oil such as almond or soya, for most of them are fairly strong and if rubbed in neat, may cause an irritation. They are also tremendously helpful for treating burns and cuts, and in other instances when the integrity of the skin is damaged. They not only reduce the possibility of infection but also stimulate the regeneration of new skin cells and so encourage the wound to heal.

Skin also acts like a mirror, reflecting the internal health of the body. In days gone by a soft, flawless skin of milky paleness was thought of as the height of beauty, prized by women and much admired by men; nowadays we know that a vital, glowing, healthy – not pale – skin also means a healthy body. Conditions such as cutaneous irritation, eczema and skin lesions all point to the fact that something is amiss, and action should be taken to treat the cause of such problems.

After the skin has taken up essential oils, the oils are eliminated through the normal channels, in the exhaled air, sweat, urine and faeces, and the organs and glands through which they pass benefit from their presence.

Through Massage

The best and most effective way to treat with essential oils is by massage. This could be as professional or as perfunctory as you like, but the rubbing action will activate the nerve endings and stimulate the circulation of blood to the surface of the skin – and thereby ease the entry of the oils. And massage is such a relaxant anyway.

Even if correctly applied, essential oils will only be taken up by the skin for a period of about seven to ten minutes, and will not be absorbed well if applied when the body is eliminating – when sweating through anxiety or heat, for instance, or after exercise. And their efficiency in penetrating the skin and reaching the other organs also depends very much on the individual. A large amount of subcutaneous fat will impede their passage, as will water retention and poor circulation.

In the Bath

Another effective way of treating with essential oils is to add a few drops to a warm bath. Make sure the room is warm, and that the door and window are closed to keep in the vapours. Immerse your body completely for at least ten minutes, relax and breathe deeply. A certain quantity of odoriferous molecules will penetrate the skin, whilst others will stimulate the nerve endings of the olfactory organ in the nose in the same way as they do when inhaled as a vapour.

These nerve endings are an extension of the limbic portion of the brain which is responsible for governing our feelings of pleasure, contentment and well-being, as well as our appetite, thirst, and sexual behaviour. They also connect with another part of the brain called the hypothalamus which in turn sends chemical messages to the pituitary gland, often referred to as the master gland, as it controls every other endocrine gland in the body (the thyroid, adrenals and ovaries, etc). So, by this indirect route, the essential oils can also exert a powerful influence over the hormonal secretions from the glands, helping to stimulate an underactive organ or soothe an agitated one, so as to re-establish harmonious functioning. The most familiar example of this is the digestive juices starting to flow when the odour of cooking food is detected. Also, via the brain, odoriferous molecules can influence the autonomic nervous system, having either a stimulatory or a soothing effect on our body and mind.

In the same way as they pass through the skin, these volatile substances also diffused from the lungs into the bloodstream and are carried around the body. Other compounds such as the lead in petrol fumes find their way into the blood in the same fashion, but in contrast this toxic mineral has a highly deleterious effect on the brain and other tissues, altering behavioural patterns and learning abilities in children, whilst giving rise to headaches, fatigue, irritability and a wealth of other niggling ailments in adults.

As a Vapour

Obviously the vapours of essential oils are inhaled while sitting in a bath with added oils, or when massaging or being massaged with oils. A more direct method of inhalation is to add a few drops to a bowl of hot water. Lean over the bowl, about 22.5 cm (9 inches) from the water, with a towel enclosing both your head and the bowl, and inhale.

In Food or Drink

Essential oils can also be taken internally, in the form of tisanes or teas made from flowers or leaves, and as the herbs and spices with which we cook.

The essential oils present in the petals and leaves of herbs and other plants can be absorbed by the cells that line the stomach and intestines and from there they enter the bloodstream and lymph fluid and circulate around the body. At the same time they actually aid the proper digestion of foods. Some essential oils are rich in certain vitamins – rose and neroli, for example, contain vitamin C, whilst most others have a fair proportion of vitamins A, E and D – so they possess nutritive as well as therapeutic properties.

But I must stress that it is exceedingly dangerous to take essential oils undiluted by mouth as they are very concentrated and will have powerful and sometimes disastrous effects. Occasionally I will prescribe them myself, but even then I would only use those that have had the terpenes (which can irritate the stomach lining) removed, and I would never advise anyone to take pure essential oils internally themselves.

TREATING ILLNESSES

There are a few items which are necessary – or useful – for treating with essential oils. They are:

– a china bowl
– a dropper for measuring out the oils
– a steel or enamel saucepan
– a few small square towels (babies' nappies are ideal)
– some small amber-coloured glass bottles with screw caps in which to keep the prepared oils (capacity about 30 ml or 1 fl. oz)
– a teaspoon, a tablespoon and an eggcup.

Measurements in the remedies for various ailments throughout the book are my recommended guidelines. As most of the measured doses of oil are drops, a dropper *is* necessary, but the quantity of the oil in which the essential oils are mixed is not so vital, so I have used teaspoons, tablespoons and the less usual eggcup. Most eggcups measure about 30 ml, which is approximately 1 fl. oz.

Flu and Colds

Many of the symptoms of colds and flu are the same – sneezing, feverishness, aching limbs, sore throat, catarrh and sinusitis. Although flu is invariably initiated by a filtrant virus, just what brings on a cold still remains rather a mystery.

As you lose your sense of smell with either a cold or flu, it is important to shake them off as quickly as possible. My advice is to rest, stay away from work for a few days until you have recovered, and to take the following steps.

When the first symptoms appear, rub your chest, sinus areas (around the eyes and nose) and inside your nostrils with either of the following mixtures.

1 drop of eucalyptus
1 drop of clove
1 drop of pine
1 eggcup of almond or any other 'cold pressed' vegetable oil

Mix all together, and decant into a glass bottle.

1 drop of cinnamon
1 drop of niaouli
1 drop of lemon
1 eggcup of vegetable oil

Mix all together and bottle.

If you have a fever, which is usually a good sign because it is the body's way of fighting off the virus, your body will be using a good deal of energy. Eating foods which are difficult to digest saps the available energy and you would be wisest to eat very little for the first two days; thereafter eat fresh fruit, which helps the cleansing process, and natural yoghurt sprinkled with wheatgerm and sweetened with honey.

Your body will also lose water through sweating and will

shed the minerals sodium and potassium, which need to be replaced. Make this tisane, which is rich in these nutrients.

1 stick of cinnamon
2 cloves
2 sprigs of fresh thyme (3 pinches dried)
1 litre (2 pints) water

Mix everything in a saucepan and boil for 2 minutes, then leave to infuse, covered with a clean cloth, for 5 minutes. Strain and drink throughout the day interpersed with fresh lemon juice mixed with mineral water and honey or fructose (fruit sugar). Keep the tisane in a jug in the fridge for no more than 2 days.

For inhaling, which will help to relieve the congestion and dispel catarrh, to a bowl of hot water (not boiling, just hand hot), add 4 drops of the following mixture.

1 drop of eucalyptus
1 drop of niaouli
1 drop of pine
1 eggcup of almond or other oil

Inhale for at least 5–10 minutes with a towel over your head to seal in the vapours four or five times a day at regular intervals. Alternatively, take two or more warm/hot baths (morning and evening), adding 2 drops of eucalyptus and 2 drops of niaouli while it is running. Soak for 10 minutes, then dry yourself vigorously, wrap up in a warm dressing gown, go back to bed and drink some of the tisane. Whilst you are bathing keep the bathroom door closed to seal in the vapours and make sure that the room is pre-heated.

You could also sprinkle a few drops of the inhaling oil on a cotton handkerchief and inhale throughout the day.

Once the symptoms have cleared, keep using the essences for another ten days, adding them to your bath, rubbing them into your chest, drinking the tisane once a day, taking plenty of lemon and other freshly squeezed juices to build up your resistance; otherwise you will only fall ill again.

To guard against colds and flu, especially if working in an office with other people who are suffering, mix up the following ingredients and decant into a glass bottle.

1 drop of eucalyptus
1 drop of clove
1 drop of pine
1 drop of cinnamon
1 drop of niaouli
2 eggcups of almond or other oil

To fumigate your room sprinkle a few drops of this mixture on a ball of lightly dampened cotton wool and place on the radiator, or mix a few drops of the essences pine, clove, eucalyptus and cinnamon minus the oil, in water and decant into an atomiser to spray your room.

You can also rub some of the essences in oil into your chest and around your nose for added protection.

Sore Throat

This often accompanies flu or a cold and can be very uncomfortable. To ease the pain, gargle with either of the following (about 6 times a day).

1. To cooled, boiled water add honey and freshly squeezed juice of half a lemon.
2. Boil a handful of dried rose petals in 1 litre (2 pints) of water for 2 minutes and then leave to infuse for 5 minutes. When just warm add 1 drop of lemon essential oil or the juice of 1 lemon.

You could also drink either of these mixtures six times a day for a couple of days and thereafter twice a day.

Earache

Earache, when associated with flu or a cold, is frequently

brought on by the spreading of the infection in the nose and throat. Symptoms include not only sore ears, but diminished hearing and feverishness as well.

To help fight the infection, warm some almond oil in a cup near the radiator and add either a crushed clove of garlic or a teaspoon of finely chopped onion and allow to steep for a couple of hours. Before going to bed, put a few drops into your eardrum using the dropper, sealing in the oil with a small ball of cotton wool and leave it in overnight.

Clean around the outside of the ear with 2 drops of clove mixed with an eggcup of soya oil to help prevent infection – and also to counteract the smell of the garlic or onion!

Tonsillitis

This affliction is caused by inflammation of the tonsils, which become painful and swollen, making it hard to swallow, and it is sometimes accompanied by other symptoms such as a cough, headache, earache, fever, chills, nausea, nasal obstruction and discharge.

To fight the infection gargle with the same remedies recommended for a sore throat. In addition, drink plenty of cool fresh pineapple juice which helps to fluidify the mucus, as well as vitamin C-rich rosehip tea and/or fresh lemon juice mixed with mineral water, sweetened with honey if desired.

A marvellous way of soothing the discomfort is to suck ice cubes made with boiled water mixed with fresh lemon and pineapple juice – as many as you like throughout the day.

Bronchitis

Bronchitis is often triggered off by a bacterial or viral infection, and is the inflammation of the air passages in the lungs. It can be either acute or chronic. Bad posture, lack of exercise and nervous tension can all make you more susceptible to suffering from bronchitis because they reduce the ability of your lungs to work to their full capacity. A poor diet which fails to supply your body with sufficient quantities of nutrients needed to help you fight off the infection can also be a contributory factor, as can tobacco smoke.

The natural mucus produced to lubricate the respiratory and nasal passages contains a natural antibiotic, and it is also rich in lactic acid which promotes the growth of beneficial ones in check. Tobacco smoke and other pollutants in the air, like sulphur dioxide, can upset the balance of these bacteria, thus making you more susceptible to bronchial infections; they can also irritate the condition once it has taken a hold, so avoid them whenever possible.

In an attempt to expel the mucus manufactured by the inflamed bronchial tubes we cough, and for this reason bronchitis is often a chesty complaint. An elevated temperature which makes you feverish, chest pains and even an irritation between the shoulder blades can also go hand in hand with bronchitis. It is important to steer clear of cold damp air which acts as an irritant, as does direct heat from, say, a radiator or open fire.

For long-term prevention of bronchitis add garlic and onions (raw whenever possible) to your food and use them liberally in your cooking. For added protection and for treatment, take 2–4 garlic perles daily especially during the winter months. For children, it is a good idea to add 3 drops of tincture of iodine to a mixture of milk and honey which should be taken every day for three months.

During a bout of bronchitis mix together the following:

1 drop of *eucalyptus*
1 drop of *hyssop*
1 drop of *pine*
1 eggcup of *almond or other oil*

Add 10 drops of this to your bath, or inhale everyday by adding 4 drops to a bowl of hand-hot water. Breathe in the fumes with your head covered by a towel.

Also rub the mixture into your chest every morning and in the evening before going to bed.

In the case of acute bronchitis, make a tea by boiling 5 cloves and 6 eucalyptus leaves in water for 2 minutes. Leave to steep for at least 5 minutes and then strain and add the juice of half a freshly squeezed lemon.

Drink plenty of fresh pineapple and lemon juice, rose-petal and rosehip tea, sweetened with honey if desired, as often as you can.

Sinusitis

This condition is caused by the inflammation of the sinus passages, and the symptoms include nasal congestion, mucus discharge, fatigue headaches, and earache, pain around the eyes, a mild fever and cough. Sinusitis often makes an appearance after you have had a cold or tonsillitis, but can also be triggered off by a deficiency of vitamin A and heavy smoking. Poor mouth hygiene and cold, damp weather do not help either. The best safeguard is to take 2–4 capsules of cod-liver or halibut oil a day for a period of three months. Whilst suffering, inhale 3 drops of the following mixture in a bowl of hot water.

1 drop of niaouli
1 drop of eucalyptus
1 drop of pine
1 eggcup of almond oil

You can also add about 10 drops of this oil to your bath and rub it into your chest and sinus area, keeping this treatment up for two months if you really want your sinusitis to clear for good.

Arthritis and Rheumatism

Arthritis is an inflammation which afflicts the joints and gives rise to a good deal of pain and stiffness. Sometimes the quantity of synovial fluid – which lubricates the joints – increases, which causes swelling and inhibits freedom of movement. There are two different kinds of arthritis – osteoarthritis and rheumatoid arthritis – and they often appear after injury, physical over-exertion or intense emotional stress.

Rheumatism is also an inflammatory condition, which affects the soft tissues, ligaments, tendons and muscles that surround and are attached to the joints. Not so long ago it was blamed on a virus, but this is no longer thought to be the case as no such organism has yet been isolated or identified. Various different varieties of rheumatism include fibrositis, a form of muscular rheumatism, and neuritis, which affects the nerves and the myelin sheath surrounding them – sciatica is a form of neuritis involving the sciatic nerve which runs from the back of the thigh, down the inside of the leg to the ankle. Lumbago is a pain in the lumbar region of the spine which effectively puts you out of action. Frozen shoulder and tennis elbow also fall into this category.

Joint and soft tissue problems are a major cause of arthritis and rheumatism, but poorly functioning kidneys and a diet which fails to supply the minerals, particularly calcium and magnesium (needed to form the lubricant synovial fluid) also predispose you towards these illnesses.

Arthritis Treatment

1 drop of thyme
1 drop of rosemary
1 drop of juniper
1 drop of sassafras
1 eggcup of almond oil

Mix all together and bottle. Apply and rub the oil into the affected area and wrap in a hot, damp towel afterwards. Try to do this four times a day.

Rheumatism Treatment

2 drops of oregano
1 drop of juniper berry
2 drops of rosemary
1 eggcup of almond oil

Mix together and bottle. As for arthritis, rub the oil into the affected area four times a day if possible. This is also good for sciatica, tennis elbow, lumbago and so forth.

Hayfever

Hayfever afflicts many people during the spring and summer months. Sufferers are usually people who have allergic tendencies and they react to any number of pollens, but more commonly to grass. Hayfever is characterised by an irritation of the membranes of the eyes and nasal passages which results in a running nose similar to that brought on by a cold, an itchy nose, eyes and throat, and is often accompanied by violent sneezing and/or a cough. Often the body tissues swell slightly because the histamine released during an allergic reaction causes them to retain water, and the skin tends to feel itchy as well.

Other airborne allergens such as dust, certain smells, moulds and chemical pollutants can invoke similar symptoms. Bad breathing habits can make you more susceptible to hayfever as well, because the body is deprived of oxygen, thus allowing the level of carbon dioxide in the blood to rise.

Poor posture, smoking and constipation prevent the body from eliminating the toxic wastes produced during metabolic processes, so they are thrown off in the form of catarrh and a heavy mucus in the alimentary tract. Milk and cheese encourage their formation and should be avoided by hayfever sufferers and replaced by substitutes like soya milk.

TREATMENT

Take ¼ teaspoon of pollen granules each day, as a very small quantity appears to be highly beneficial. Garlic is also good for hayfever and other respiratory disorders, so add it to your food or take garlic perles daily.

Make a tisane to drink during an attack by boiling pine needles and eucalyptus leaves, a pinch of each in 500 ml (a scant pint) of water. Drink plenty of rosehip tea, rich in Vitamin C, a nutrient that is used up during an attack.

For sore, itchy eyes, apply compresses soaked in either cornflower, camomile or marigold infusions.

Asthma

Asthma is a respiratory problem which often goes hand in hand with bronchitis, nervous disorders and hayfever, and also tends to afflict people of a nervous disposition. During an attack sufferers have great difficulty in breathing and often feel a sense of suffocation, the chest feels tight and heavy, and he or she has to cough to get rid of the mucus.

Sufferers should avoid stimulants such as tea, chocolate and coffee whenever possible and replace them with herbal tisanes. Take eucalyptus and thyme together, or others like passiflora (passion flower), camomile, valerian and aniseed.

It is not wise to inhale the vapours of essential oils as asthma sufferers are allergy-prone people and may react to odoriferous substances, perhaps actually worsening an attack.

Halitosis

Halitosis can be caused by any number of things (see page 38), but simply to make your mouth taste sweeter, and your breath smell fresher, make this mouthwash. To a cup or glass of cooled, boiled water add 1 drop of myrrh essence and use for gargling.

Pyorrhoea

This is a condition whereby the gums become infected and you will need to mouthwash every day. The same recipe could also be used for mouth sores or an ulcerated throat, or when teeth have been extracted.

Boil a handful of sage leaves in 1 litre (2 pints) of water for 2 minutes, then infuse for 5 minutes. Add a drop of essential oil of myrrh and brush the gums gently with a soft, silk brush.

Piles or haemorrhoids

Bathe the affected area with very cold water and then apply a mixture of 1 drop of myrrh, 1 drop of cypress, and 3 teaspoons of soya oil.

CHAPTER FIVE

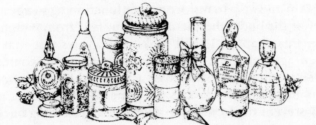

Aromatherapy and Beauty

True beauty is an expression of inner health, youthfulness and sexuality, so nothing is more attractive than a fresh, flawless complexion that literally glows with vitality. Barefaced is best, and no-one should have to rely on cosmetic coverage, as women did even a decade ago, to disguise a less than perfect skin.

Women have been attempting to beautify their skin from the outside since antiquity, by applying various weird and wonderful concoctions. And within the last fifty years, there has been a phenomenal growth in the number of skin-care products on the market, with women spending more and more money on such treatments for the face. The problem is that the changes such creams can bring about are minimal, for they only work superficially. The real nature of skin is determined by *inner* health, and many women have less than perfect skins because of the battle their bodies wage continually with the hectic twentieth-century lifestyle: fast convenience foods, stress, lack of exercise, and industrial pollutants, all these, and more work to undermine the condition of the skin.

Queen Hatshepsut, the first woman pharaoh of Egypt, knew more about beauty than most, and was years ahead of her time in realising that aromatherapy skin treatments are unlike any others. Because essential oils can penetrate the skin and help to restore proper functioning to any ailing part of the body, they actually beautify it from within.

In this chapter, I shall look at the ways essential oils, when applied daily, can bring out the best in your skin, correct minor imbalances such as oiliness and dryness, treat troubling skin disorders such as acne, psoriasis and eczema, and prevent the formation of wrinkles by holding back the ageing process.

THE FACE

To understand how essential oils can work in this way, it is important to know in more detail than defined before about the structure and functions of the skin.

The outer epidermis consists of many layers of skin cells. New, round, plump ones are produced at the basal layer and travel up towards the surface of the skin, losing their moisture and becoming flatter all the while, until they are shed as dead skin cells. By the time they are ready to be shed, in a process known as exfoliation, these cells are rich in a protein called keratin, the same stuff of which fingernails are composed, so they are quite brittle and scaly. On average, it takes about 120 days for newly formed cells to move up to the skin surface and die. The time, however, varies according to the individual, the individual's age, and several other factors.

The epidermis rests on the inner dermis, which acts rather like a cushion, giving strength and support as well as contour to the skin. Within the dermis we find an ordered network of tough collagen fibres, made from proteinaceous material, which lie in a ground substance forming what is known as connective tissue. Also present are elastin fibres which give skin pliancy and stretchability rather than strength. A young, healthy skin has the capacity to increase its size by 50 per cent due to these elastic properties, but this function diminishes with age.

The dermis is richly supplied by many small capillaries which bring oxygen and other vital nutrients to the skin cells and carry away the toxic waste products. It is also well endowed with nerve endings which surround the hair follicles and form a kind of sensory apparatus, transmitting messages from the skin surface concerning temperature, touch and pain, so as to invoke the appropriate response.

Sebaceous glands are also present in the dermis, but they open to the surface at pores located in the epidermis. These glands produce the oily substance called sebum, whose function is to lubricate the skin and to seal moisture in the cells. Their activity determines whether your skin is normal, oily or dry.

In turn, your skin type is influenced genetically, and if you have fair hair, you are more likely to have pale, and perhaps rather delicate, skin than someone who is dark.

So it is quite obvious, if you want your skin to look its best, you should always care for it appropriately.

Normal Skin

People with normal skin are lucky as they tend to have few problems. At the same time, it still needs to be well looked after to keep it supple and ensure that the sebaceous secretions maintain their equilibrium: many things, such as tiredness, illness, rapid weight loss, smoking and drinking, can disrupt this fine balance. To test whether your skin is normal or not, close your eyes and place your index finger on your forehead. If it feels slightly damp, not oily, then it is normal.

To care for your skin, wash with an acid or pH balanced soap in warm water, finishing with a tonic of rose tea, and use a facial oil every day. Make your own by adding 1 drop of rose and 1 drop of camomile essential oil to 3–4 teaspoons of almond oil. Apply this oil every morning and evening.

A good massage will not only help the absorption of the essential oils, but will also stimulate the circulation, encouraging the delivery of fresh blood to the skin cells. Make circular movements with your fingers around the sinus area, over the cheeks and chin, scissor across the forehead and stroke up the neck, back and front.

Use a face mask once a week to help refine the pores. To make your own rose and oatmeal mask, place a cup of oatmeal into a mixing bowl and add boiling water little by little. Mix to a thick paste. Add 1 drop of rose essence and a little almond or soya oil to stop it drying out. You could also make two poultices, one for the forehead and cheeks, and another for the chin and neck. Make two 'sandwiches' with four squares of gauze and some of the oatmeal mix. Apply the poultices to the face, at the same time covering the eyes with cotton wool pads soaked in rose water. Relax and leave for 10 minutes.

Even a normal skin can look dull and lifeless at times, so to improve its colour, work to stimulate the circulation by massage, washing firstly with warm-hot water and then with cold, and by taking plenty of exercise. Eat plenty of foods rich in Vitamins C, A and the entire B complex, for they are excellent skin nourishers.

Oily Skin

During adolescence, when the hormones are undergoing dramatic changes, it is very common for the sebaceous glands to become overactive, and cause a condition known as seborrhoea. The skin looks shiny, the pores are often enlarged, and the skin is more likely to suffer from blackheads and spots.

It is fairly easy to recognise an oily skin: place a piece of blotting paper or fine greaseproof paper on different areas of the skin, and the stains left will give an indication as to just how severe the condition is. Normally, it is only people who live in hot countries and eat spicy foods that have a very bad problem, as both these things provoke the already overactive glands into producing even more oil.

Indeed, if your skin has a tendency towards oiliness, it is worth knowing that it can be made worse by stimulants such as tea, coffee, and the nicotine in cigarettes, by a diet rich in fatty foods (especially meats like pork and lamb), by sugar and foods containing it such as cakes, sweets and biscuits and, on the other hand, by emotional upsets like worry, anxiety, fear and anger.

People who suffer from constipation often have oily skin, so it is important to eat plenty of natural fibre or roughage which is found in raw fruits and vegetables, pulses, legumes, and whole grains.

Certain essential oils can be extremely helpful in treating oily skin, as they have a balancing influence and reduce the activity of the sebaceous glands, so helping the skin to behave as if it were normal.

TREATMENT
Wash the face with a mild, acid balanced soap and cool water. Never use a milky cleanser or cream which will leave an unwanted film of grease on the skin. Rinse with warm and then cold water, and finally dampen the skin with cotton wool soaked in a diluted solution of witch-hazel.

Make a facial oil by adding 1 drop of juniper and 1 drop of geranium to 2 teaspoons of soya or jojoba oil. Pour some of this into the palm of your hand and gently massage it into your skin. Once the first application has been absorbed, add another. To aid the penetration of the essences soak a small towel in boiling water, and when it has cooled to hand-hot temperature, wring it out and cover the face as if it were a compress.

Once a week give your face a sauna, by adding 1 drop of juniper and 1 drop of geranium to a bowl of hot water and steaming your face with the vapours.

Dry Skin

Dry skin results from an inability of the sebaceous glands to produce the quantity of oil needed to prevent the skin from losing moisture. As a consequence it feels taut, as if tightly stretched across the face, and tends to suffer from flakiness. A dry skin is less supple than a normal one, which makes it more prone to fine surface lines, and so it is likely to age prematurely. It is also highly sensitive, and easily irritated by harsh detergents and cosmetics, becoming red and blotchy.

Many things can exacerbate the dry skin condition and even make an otherwise normal skin become dehydrated. Internal causes are illness, a diet deficient in vital nutrients (especially vitamin F, the essential fatty acids), sudden and rapid weight loss, taking drugs such as antibiotics and tranquillisers, and drinking too much alcohol. External environmental hazards take the form of direct sunlight (and sunbeds), central heating, and icy wintry winds.

TREATMENT
A skin that feels tight should never be washed more than once a week, and even then only with a very mild soap. For everyday cleansing make a tonic by steeping camomile flowers in boiling water (or you can use a camomile tea bag instead). When this infusion has cooled, add a few drops of jojoba oil, and wash your face with it.

A marvellously effective facial oil can be made for dry skin by mixing 4–5 teaspoons of almond oil with 2–2½ teaspoons of castor oil (or 2 parts almond to 1 part castor), adding 1 capsule (or ¼ teaspoon) of cod-liver oil, 1 drop of calendula, 1 drop of hyssop, and 1 teaspoon of wheatgerm oil. Massage into the skin with very light stroking movements only, for dry skin tends to be very delicate and may become irritated with rough handling. Leave the oil on for 10 minutes, applying a warm compress which has been soaked in either rose water or linden tea.

When the skin improves you can use an oil made from almond oil and essences alone.

Combination Skin

This is a skin that has oily and dry patches, and may be slightly affected by the change of seasons. Most of the time you can treat it as if it were normal, but if the sebaceous glands of the so-called centre panel – the nose, forehead, and chin – flare up, which they may do in periods of stress or just before a period, it is advisable to treat the area with the facial oil prescribed for an oily skin.

Puffiness

When the tissues of the body become laden with water, the face often takes on a puffy or swollen appearance, especially just under the eyes. This often happens just before menstruation, when women are particularly prone to water retention, or it can come on after an illness, if you are taking drugs, or if you have an allergic reaction which irritates the sinuses like hayfever. Sometimes it is a sign that the kidneys are not eliminating as well as they might, or that undigested food has been absorbed into the bloodstream.

To reduce the oedema, wash the skin with a gentle soap, then rinse in cold water. Make up some camomile tea by boiling a pinch of dried flowers in 500 ml (a scant pint) of water, and soak a compress of gauze in it. Apply this to the skin – or you could simply use a camomile tea bag.

Make a face oil by adding 1 drop of sandalwood and 1 drop of geranium or 1 drop of cypress and 1 drop of sandalwood to 2 teaspoons of cold pressed almond oil.

Massage into the face, applying deep pressure around the sinus area and the mouth. Then reapply a camomile compress and leave for 5–10 minutes to help the essential oils penetrate the skin.

Never apply a thick eye cream at night, for this will make them even puffier, and as far as food is concerned, stay away from salt and sugar, especially if prone to pre-menstrual water retention, for they encourage this problem, particularly salt.

Broken Capillaries

This is the Anglo-Saxon woman's complaint, for it afflicts fair, delicate skins which also tend to burn in the sun. It is characterised by the appearance of fine, red spider veins on the cheeks which make them look ruddy. Often the capillaries are not actually broken, just weak and transparent, so that the blood shows through them.

It is important to avoid drinking stimulants such as tea, coffee and chocolate as well as alcohol which cause the capillaries to dilate; the skin must also be protected from direct sunlight and icy winds. It is advisable not to take over-strenuous exercise. Never wash your face with hot water or use a facial sauna if you suffer from broken capillaries, and avoid taking hot baths.

Use a cool compress of parsley tea on the face daily: boil 3 sprigs of fresh parsley in 500 ml (a scant pint) of water for 2 minutes and then leave to steep for 5 minutes; add a drop of rose and a drop of marigold, and leave to cool.

Massage the face very gently with a facial oil made from a mixture of 1 drop of parsley, 1 drop of camomile, 2 teaspoons of soya oil and 1 teaspoon of wheatgerm oil. If you use this oil every day, within a few months you will notice that the high colouring has faded, for the essential oils have the ability not only to drain the capillaries, but also to strengthen them. Eating foods rich in bioflavinoids and

Vitamin C, both vital to capillary health – such as oranges, grapefruit and lemons – is also advisable if you are prone to this problem.

SKIN PROBLEMS

The skin is a mirror of body health, and the nature of skin is greatly influenced by changes that take place from within, far more so than by any cream applied to the surface. For this reason any skin problem should be regarded as an indication that your health is not what it could be, and if treatment is to be successful, you have to consider the body as a whole, not just from a superficial angle. A skin problem may be the result of many years of bad eating habits, of acute emotional anxiety, of a biochemical disorder such as hyperglycaemia or diabetes, or of a reaction to aerosol sprays, antibiotics or other drugs – even to skin-care products themselves.

The skin is an organ with many different functions. It helps to maintain constant body temperature by shedding excess heat in the form of water, as sweat that cools as it evaporates on the surface of the skin. In this way it also eliminates toxins or unwanted waste products from the body. By blocking up these natural eliminating channels with the use of anti-perspirants and heavy face make-up the toxins can actually build up in layers within the skin, which may eventually be expelled in the form of spots and pimples. Their appearance is often a clear sign that the cleansing organs of the body, the liver and kidneys primarily, are not working properly to eliminate the wastes; the skin is thus called upon to act as a sort of dumping ground to relieve the body of these unwanted substances. Invariably once the liver and kidneys are back to normal, the condition of the skin rapidly improves.

Conditions such as eczema are often a symptom of an

internal illness or disorder, and act as a means through which the body can discharge its affliction. Sometimes by curing the eczema with drugs you remove this eliminative pathway, so the problem builds up inside and may erupt, perhaps years later. You can treat the symptoms gently and safely with essential oils, knowing that you will not be causing any damage.

Acne

Acne is a disorder of the sebaceous or oil-secreting glands of the skin, which gives rise to enlarged pores, blackheads, pimples and pustules. It tends to afflict areas of the skin where these glands are found in abundance – the face and back, for instance. The condition is initiated by an over-production of oil which is too copious for the skin to handle, so it ends up looking greasy. At the same time it blocks up the pores making them appear larger than they actually are, and results in the formation of blackheads. If the sebum in these clogged pores becomes infected by a bacterium such as staphylococcus, which is ever-present on the surface of the skin, spots form that may ultimately turn into unsightly boils. The skin and spots are usually inflamed, and often quite painful to touch.

Sebum secretion actually begins within the uterus, which is why some babies can be born with an oily skin, but this usually disappears within two months, and is no indication that the child will develop acne in later life. Acne flares up most during the pubescent years, afflicting many adolescents and young adults. Sometimes it corrects itself after the mid-twenties and sometimes it does not subside again until after middle age. One of the underlying causes of this over-production of sebum is thought to be a glandular disorder which gives rise to hormonal imbalance, usually characterised by a predominance of male hormones or androgens. The fact that the severity of this condition changes throughout the menstrual cycle reinforces the idea that the sex hormones are involved, for acne tends to flare up about a week before a woman is due to begin her period. Indeed, even women with good skins may find they develop a few pimples around this time.

Stress and anxiety, both of which interfere with the levels of hormones in the body, also spell trouble for acne sufferers, and a vicious circle can often be set into motion with worry giving rise to more spots and these causing further worry.

Acne sufferers can invariably be helped by exercise, especially outdoors, and by paying careful attention to their diet. Well-balanced meals concentrating on foods rich in vitamins A, B1, B2 and B6, plus plenty of fresh fruit and vegetables, are vital. Fatty foods such as pork and lamb should be avoided, as should stimulants like tea, coffee, alcohol and cigarettes which only aggravate the acne condition: they should be replaced by mineral water, tisanes and, in small quantities, fresh fruit juices diluted with water.

Essential oils can go a long way towards helping an acne skin become healthy again. They can banish the spots, heal up the scars and reduce the inflammation that make this condition so unpleasant. Most of the young people who come and see me at my practice with this problem have tried antibiotics and all the other drugs on the market but to no avail.

One such client, very typical of acne sufferers, is a young girl who had been on strong antibiotics for six years, so long that her skin was no longer responding; the boils were still appearing, whilst the scars were red and inflamed. She had recently lost her job and felt that her acne had been responsible, because it was so unattractive. She was very depressed, her self-confidence and self-esteem were low, and she desperately needed help.

I explained that a natural cure would be a lengthy process

and she could not expect overnight results. In fact it might be a year before substantial improvements could be seen. She accepted this and had some treatments. I discovered that the antibiotics had not helped, in addition to which she admitted to drinking alcohol and coffee freely, and replacing her meals with nutritionally inadequate snacks. She carried on using the oils at home and I kept a check on her diet. It was three months before there was any improvement, but small patches of her facial skin began to clear and the scars healed. One and a half years later she has a beautiful skin, and it is difficult to tell that she ever suffered from such a problem.

Another success story, and luckily there have been many, is that of a seventeen-year-old boy who had been suffering from acne for four years. The antibiotics he had been taking had worked for about three months before becoming ineffectual, which led to even stronger ones being prescribed. When I saw him the acne was so advanced that his face was swollen and marred by abscesses. He only came to see me once because he lived so far away, but I gave him a cleanser, oil and cream to use together with pure essences which could be applied undiluted to the infected spots. After a few months patches of healthy skin started to appear, and nine months following his visit he sent me a photograph, and I found it difficult to believe it was the same person. His skin was healthy-looking and clear except for the odd pimple from which all teenagers occasionally suffer, and the treatment has stood the test of time.

TREATMENT

All too often people with acne resort to using powerful detergents and alcoholic astringents to remove every trace of oil. The skin *needs* a certain amount of oil for lubrication and protection, however, so it is not long before the sebaceous glands respond by producing even more oil, so exacerbating the problem. Although people are wary of using an oil on an already oily skin, it should be remembered that essential oils are actually made up of molecules such as alcohols, phenols, and terpenes and because they are quickly absorbed, little trace of oil is actually left on the skin. They not only help to restore equilibrium to the sebaceous glands but also keep the bacteria in check because of their natural antibiotic properties. They also act at a much deeper level on the glands to correct the hormonal imbalances, but they do take time to work, and you have to persevere.

Treatment involves cleansing, steaming, applying a facial oil to improve the general condition of the skin, and pure essences to treat the spots themselves.

CLEANSING
Wash the skin with an *unscented* pH balanced or acid soap, in hot water, and rinse thoroughly in cold. You can always use mineral or distilled water if you are concerned about dehydrating effects.

Make an astringent by boiling a sprig of fresh thyme or, a pinch of dried, in 2 cups of water for 2 minutes, then leave to infuse for 5 minutes. Add the juice of half a lemon and rinse the skin with this solution, two to three times a day. Men should use it after shaving.

You can make a compress by soaking a piece of gauze in this solution, wringing out the excess and covering the face with it for 5 minutes. This is a good treatment before going out for the evening.

FACIAL SAUNA
This should be done three or four times a week when the acne is severe, and reduced to once a week when it begins to improve. Boil a kettle of water and wait until it has cooled to hand-hot temperature (about 38°C/100°F), not scalding. Pour into a bowl and add:

1 drop of lavender
1 drop of camomile
1 drop of petitgrain

If the condition is very acute you could mix together any two of the following essences instead: neroli, juniper, lavender or clove. In both cases, hold your face over the bowl with a towel enclosing the bowl and your head, and let the vapours work on your skin.

FACIAL OILS
To be used morning and evening after cleansing.

2 tablespoons of soya oil
2 drops of lavender
1 drop of camomile
1 drop of petitgrain

Mix together and keep in an amber bottle. Make two applications, the second once the oil of the first has been absorbed. To aid absorption apply hot compresses to the face 5 minutes after the second application.

PURE ESSENCES
Because of their strong antibacterial properties, undiluted essential oils – any of the ones recommended above – are useful for applying straight to the pimples and pustules on a cottonwool bud every day.

Psoriasis

Psoriasis is an unsightly condition, characterised by circular patches of dry scaly skin which are either pale pink or dark wine red in colour. It appears predominantly on the knees and elbows, and sometimes on the scalp and top of the forehead. Fortunately, it rarely appears on the face.

The reason for its sudden appearance still remains a mystery, but we do know that if someone in the family has suffered from it, there is a likelihood that you may too. It afflicts both sexes alike, and will appear at any age, but most frequently after twenty. People with fair skins such as Europeans and North Americans seem to be particularly susceptible to psoriasis, and it is rare amongst Japanese and Negro populations.

Once it strikes, psoriasis is likely to linger for a long time, and is notoriously difficult to cure. There are several different types, some of which can actually be brought on by treatment of the psoriasis with corticosteroids. Sometimes it can become so dry that the skin cracks, and this is extremely uncomfortable and painful. In the case of pustular psoriasis the skin can actually become infected.

Surprisingly perhaps, psoriasis is not infectious and there is no possibility of catching it by touching someone suffering from it.

Although psoriasis is difficult to cure, it *is* treatable, and essential oils are tremendously effective. I have helped many psoriasis sufferers who have come to the practice.

One lady, a musician, had very bad psoriasis on her hands which were cracked and sore, making it difficult for her to pursue her career. Interestingly, it did not appear until she was thirty, but her mother had been a sufferer too. I asked her never to use detergents – she should use instead a solution of soapwort, one of nature's most effective cleansers – and to rub oils into her hands and keep them on for a few hours by wearing cotton gloves. She altered her diet, including plenty of foods rich in vitamin A, took more exercise than before, and two years later she has the occasional rash on her knees, but nothing worse. Her skin has returned to normal.

Another case, a man who had psoriasis on his scalp had been given a black, sticky concoction to smear onto his affected skin by a dermatologist. This treatment helped a little, but he wasn't at all happy with it. I made him a shampoo and a special oil, which have alleviated his problem to the extent that he now absolutely swears by them.

As with all skin disorders, psoriasis points to some deep-rooted ailment, and so anything which encourages the health to deteriorate such as smoking and drinking alcohol are best avoided. The condition is also irritated by wearing polyester or nylon next to the skin, which prevents it from breathing properly, and people with psoriasis on their scalp should not wear tight-fitting hats or nylon scarves. Extremes of temperature will also aggravate it, so you should avoid sitting next to open fires and, whenever possible, stay in when it's very cold outside.

INTERNAL TREATMENT
Look for foods rich in vitamin A and lecithin. Take 2 capsules of cod-liver oil a day, or a teaspoon, and try taking 1–2 capsules of evening primrose oil which can also be very helpful. It is also a good idea to make some sage tea and drink two or more cups a day in place of coffee and tea.

EXTERNAL TREATMENT
Add an infusion of birch leaves or marigold flowers to the bath, with 2 drops of cajput together with 1 drop of thyme, or 2 drops of calendula plus 1 drop of oregano.

Instead of soap, wash with a solution of soapwort made by boiling about 5 g (a scant ¼ oz) of soapwort leaves and root in 1 litre (2 pints) of water, and sponging the affected area.

After washing apply one of the following oils. Mix together with an eggcup of soya oil, either 1 teaspoon of wheatgerm oil and 1 teaspoon of castor oil, or 2 drops of calendula and 1 drop of oregano. Sometimes you have to experiment to find the right personal combination of essential oils. Always use 3 drops in total of essential oils and if the other oils are not very effective try different mixes using cajput, thyme, calendula and oregano.

Alternatively to the eggcup of soya oil, add 1 capsule of vitamin A, 2 capsules of lecithin, 1 drop of calendula and 1 drop of cajput.

FOR THE SCALP

Before shampooing, massage the scalp with an infusion of marigold flowers. Boil 4 flower heads in 500 ml (a scant pint) of water for 2 minutes, let it steep for 5 minutes, and then add the juice of half a lemon.

Alternatively you could rub in a solution of boiled birch leaves mixed with a teaspoon of cider vinegar.

Dilute your shampoo with either birch-leaf or camomile tea and rinse with a tablespoon of either lemon juice or cider vinegar.

Avoid using a hairdryer if possible, letting your hair dry naturally instead, as direct heat will only irritate the condition.

Dermatitis

Dermatitis is an inflammatory skin condition often associated with hereditary allergic tendencies – such as food allergies to dairy products and gluten – and which invariably worsens or appears for the first time when a person has suffered a severe emotional upset or is very fatigued and run down.

The symptoms are those of eczema which is characterised by blister-like skin eruptions that weep and form crusts. The skin then thickens and flakes, and the eczema patches are often pigmented differently from the rest of the skin.

Certain food, pollutants, a deficiency of the B complex vitamins can also cause dermatitis.

TREATMENT

You should increase your intake of foods rich in the B vitamins, especially vitamin B6. Supplement your diet with

2–4 capsules of evening primrose oil daily and a capsule of wheatgerm oil (rich in vitamin E). Use cold pressed soya, corn and safflower oil in your cooking and for salad dressings, as they are all rich in essential fatty acids (more commonly known as vitamin F), as people suffering from eczema are often deficient in this.

Cut down on saturated fats such as those found in meats and dairy products, substituting with fish, nuts and seeds instead.

Every day, rub into your skin an oil made from 3–4 teaspoons of soya oil, plus 2 drops of camomile and 2 drops of hyssop.

For very dry eczema, mix about 3 teaspoons of almond oil with the same quantity of castor oil, then add 1 drop of geranium and 1 drop of lavender. For very oily eczema, add 4 drops of juniper berry essential oil to the almond-castor oil mixture.

Also add to your bath 1 teaspoon of soya oil and a total of 2 drops of the appropriate essences.

AGEING

Every woman dreads the insidious appearance of wrinkles, which serve as a constant reminder of the years that are passing her by. It would be wonderful to discover an elixir which could ward off the ageing process or, even better, bring about total rejuvenation. But, unfortunately, this will never be possible, because the ageing process is biologically predetermined and no potion in the world is ever going to take wrinkles away. Essential oils, however, can do more than most to slow down their appearance.

One of the fundamental causes of ageing is the slowing down of cell division. Up until the time of birth there is a rapid multiplication of cells following the fertilisation of the female ovum by the male spermatozoa. After birth, this process gradually slows down and continues to diminish until we die, so we have very little influence over it.

This slowing-down process takes place at a different pace in each person, and certain things slow the natural biological processes down even further: these should be minimised or avoided completely if we are to stay youthful longer. The main culprits are illness, smoking, taking drugs, drinking alcohol, tea and coffee in excess, being subjected to too much stress, not taking enough exercise, and being exposed to radiation.

The quality of food you eat is also very important, for the organs should be supplied with sufficient quantities of nutrients if they are to function properly. I have seen women who have had anorexia with skins that reflect their internal malnutrition by looking twenty years older than they should.

I have also noticed that a person's attitude to life and their behaviour also affects the rate at which they age, so someone who has gathered a good deal of unhappiness in their lifetime, or who is always dissatisfied, will age far faster than a person who is enthusiastic and in love with life.

As far as the skin is concerned, dermatologists and cosmetic scientists now know that several changes take place as it ages.

Within the dermis the network of collagen and elastin fibres which lend skin its suppleness and firmness begins to alter and as a result deep wrinkles form which can never be removed. Certain things actually encourage these changes to take place, such as the UV rays of sunlight, and for this reason people who live in hot countries and do not shade their skin from the sun tend to have more wrinkles than those who protect their skin from the direct rays, or who live in more temperate climates. Other forms of radiation also accelerate the formation of these wrinkles, but the sun has the added disadvantage of making the skin feel leathery as well.

Changes also take place in the epidermis with the passage of time. As the rate of cell division slows down, the epidermis becomes thinner, and because the newly formed cells take longer to reach the surface, there is a larger proportion of flat, dehydrated, dead cells which gives the skin a dull, lifeless appearance instead of a fresh, translucent one.

Because the cells of the epidermis do not regenerate themselves as readily as they did when they were younger, it also means that the skin takes longer to heal itself after damage (a burn or cut, for example) than it did before.

All kinds of external factors, such as the climate, and the way you cleanse, protect and nourish your skin, will affect the condition of the epidermis, and looking after it properly from an early age certainly pays off in the long run.

To my mind the daily application of essential oils can go a long way towards helping the skin stay young, for they encourage the cells to regenerate themselves more efficiently. They also act on the sebaceous glands which often become underactive as we get older, making them produce sufficient oil to keep the skin lubricated, keeping it supple and less prone to wrinkling. Because essential oils penetrate the skin, they are far more active than most cosmetic products on the market. By helping to restore proper functioning to a tired or ailing organ or gland, they can actually eliminate some of the fundamental causes of age acceleration.

This facial oil will help keep a maturing skin young and supple.

3–4 teaspoons of almond oil
1 tablespoon of soya oil
1 teaspoon of wheatgerm oil
4 drops of galbanum
1 drop of Moroccan rose

Mix the oils together first, then add the essences. Massage gently into the face and neck and apply a hot compress soaked in an infusion of rose petals. Apply every evening.

Cleanse the skin with a gentle soap, never more than twice a week; the rest of the time use a rose-petal infusion which will not dry the skin in any way (whereas tap water may).

The massaging of the skin that goes hand in hand with applying the facial oils can help to improve the delivery of nutrients to and removal of waste products from the skin cells. It can also improve the muscle tone. We often tend to forget that it is the muscles underlying the skin that give our bodies shape and contour. When they contract, they cause the skin to wrinkle, and this is what gives rise to expression lines, which are fine providing the muscles relax again. However, due to tension, they often enter a steady state of contraction, and if they remain like this for a long time, they cause the formation of permanent wrinkles, usually furrows on the forehead.

Massaging helps to relax these muscles as well as tone up those that are under-exercised and have shrivelled up as a result, and which cause the skin to sag, usually around the jawline. In fact, the reason why face lifts are often so disappointing is because they gather up the sagging skin and stretch out the wrinkles, but actually do nothing to improve the underlying muscle tone which gives the skin its youthful contour.

There are many clients who came to my practice to be treated when their skin started to age eighteen years or more ago, and since then, amazingly, it has not deteriorated any further, for the essential oils have preserved their skin, keeping it as smooth and supple as ever. Some have found that their skin actually looks several years younger than it did before treatment and many who were planning to have plastic surgery found that, to their astonishment, it was no longer necessary.

My advice to anyone wishing to preserve the youthful look of their skin is, not only to use essential oils every day, but also to avoid sunbathing or staying out in the sun for any length of time: this applies particularly to those with varicose veins. Always protect your skin during the first week in strong sunlight, and build up a colour gradually, for once your skin has burned, it will become tremendously sensitive. Avoid sunlamps and sunbeds: they give out predominantly UV radiation, which may be the rays that give you a suntan but are also the ones that penetrate the dermis to disrupt the structure of the collagen and elastin fibres, resulting in the formation of deep and permanent wrinkles.

Remember that the skin on the neck is incredibly fragile, and ages more rapidly than the face, so it needs attention too. Bear in mind that it is under a good deal of strain, as it has to lend support to the weight of the head. Poor posture will affect the muscles and cause the skin to wrinkle. When applying your facial oil never forget to massage it into the back, as well as the front, of your neck, if you wish to reap the maximum benefits from it.

Hands may also help to give away your age, as they are continually exposed to the damaging elements. Protect them whenever possible and once a week apply one of the following oils.

1. *1 teaspoon castor oil*
   3–4 teaspoons almond oil
   2 drops of galbanum

2. *4–5 teaspoons of wheatgerm oil*
   1 drop of galbanum
   1 drop of rose
   1 drop of lemon

Mix together and decant into a small bottle. After

rubbing into the skin, put on a pair of cotton gloves and leave on for an hour or more. If inconvenient during the day, you could always wear them throughout the night. This oil is also an excellent treatment for dry, sun-parched feet.

THE HAIR

Most of us tend to think of hair in terms of colour, condition and style, and forget that it also serves a useful purpose in protecting the scalp from extremes of temperature and in regulating the loss of body heat from the head. Approximately 100,000 individual hairs grow from hair follicles in the scalp and they do so at a rate of about 2 cm (just under 1 inch) a month, although this varies from person to person.

In many respects hair is similar to skin because it reflects inner health. Each hair is made of the tough, stretchable protein material called keratin, manufactured by the hair follicle – the same material of which fingernails are made, and which is contained in dead skin cells. The condition of the developing hair is largely dependent upon a good supply of blood carrying adequate quantities of amino acids (the building blocks of proteins), vitamins E, C and the B complex, as well as minerals like calcium, zinc, iron and copper, to the hair follicle. Poor health, whatever its cause, can be responsible for hair that lacks lustre and life, and it probably grows unusually slowly into the bargain.

Also whilst the hair is being formed, different pigment molecules are laid down which determine the colour of the hair. Hair can turn grey early, following illness or a period of intense emotional distress, because such things interfere with the production of the pigment. A nutritionally inadequate diet is capable of doing the same thing.

Hair is *formed* from living material, but the actual hair itself, the hair that you brush, is dead, and after a period each one is shed and replaced by another. Its condition depends on good health and nutrition as above, but also on how it is treated. Many problems such as unmanageability and split ends are caused by actually abusing the hair through using the wrong shampoos and overdoing the styling.

It is important to know your hair, to recognise whether it is normal, or whether it has a tendency to oiliness or dryness. Alongside each hair lies a sebaceous gland which secretes sebum to lubricate the hair and lend it a degree of protection. If the glands are overactive, and produce more sebum than is needed, the hair becomes oily and will need more frequent washing to take away the excess. Do *not* resort to a more concentrated, oil-stripping shampoo, as this will only stimulate the glands into producing even more oil to compensate. If, on the other hand, the glands are sluggish, the hair will become dehydrated and dry, so you should avoid moisture-robbing hair dryers, heated curlers and exposure to sunlight, wind and sea water.

General Hair Care

Essential oils are extremely helpful in hair care as they have the ability to influence the sebaceous glands and normalise their functions. They are beneficial to all hair types, and leave hair smelling good too.

WASHING

If you use a mild or gentle shampoo you can wash your hair as frequently as you want – which might be every day for city dwellers and people with oily hair.

Make an infusion of one of the following herbs – camomile, rosemary, sage or nettle – and add a cupful to your shampoo to dilute it. Wash in warm water, then for the final rinse use cold distilled or purified water.

Every month treat your hair to a massage.

2 *teaspoons of soya oil*
1 *teaspoon of rum*
1 *capsule of cod-liver oil*
1 *capsule of lecithin*
2 *drops of thyme*
2 *drops of sage*

Mix all together, and massage into your hair for a few minutes. Then wrap your head in a warm towel to aid the penetration of the oils and leave on for an hour. When washing out the oil use a gentle shampoo, not diluted this time, and afterwards rinse through with either fresh lemon juice for fair hair or cider vinegar for dark to help restore manageability and shine. This treatment is particularly good for dull hair and hair that suffers from split ends.

Hair Problems

Most hair problems that are not directly caused by illness, poor diet, excess smoking, alcohol drinking and so on, can be traced back to excessive use of heated appliances, misuse of chemical treatments such as perming and colouring, and washing with over-strong detergent shampoos.

Hair Loss

Many women who come to me suffering from falling hair, which can lead to bald patches or alopecia, have invariably been maltreating their hair over long periods of time. It is also interesting to note that the problem is far more common today than it was twenty years ago, and in many cases it seems to afflict young women in their thirties. To my mind, the fact that women are subjected to large amounts of stress nowadays may encourage this disconcerting condition. It can also be caused by a hormonal upheaval, which is why pregnant women often experience hair loss.

It can often be helped by a good scalp massage and application of the oil treatment prescribed for normal hair.

DANDRUFF

This is a very common problem, caused by the shedding of matured unwanted skin cells and wastes from the scalp. Like alopecia, it is often linked to emotional upsets, hormonal imbalance, poor eating habits, excessive use of chemicals on the hair, and by not rinsing the hair properly. Dandruff sufferers need a well balanced diet rich in foods containing the B complex vitamins, vitamin A, and minerals, particularly zinc. Useful supplements are cod-liver oil and kelp (seaweed).

An effective, natural way of combatting dandruff is to apply pre-shampooing lotions to the scalp.

1. *50 g (2 oz) sage*
   500 ml (a scant pint) boiling water
   2 drops essential oil of sage
   2 drops essential oil of thyme
   Make an infusion by boiling the sage leaves in the water for 2 minutes, then leave to infuse for 5 minutes. Add the essential oils.

2. *3 nasturtium heads*
   500 ml (a scant pint) boiling water
   250 ml (a scant ½ pint) rum
   4 drops essential oil of rosemary
   Boil the nasturtium heads in the water for 2 minutes, then infuse for 5 minutes. Add 1 cup of this tea to the rum, and add the rosemary oil.

Rub either of these solutions into the scalp four times a week, at least, before shampooing. Then wash the hair with a shampoo made by mixing one-third shampoo and two-thirds sage infusion together, with 1 drop of sage oil. An alternative is one-third shampoo and two-thirds nasturtium tea plus 1 drop of thyme. Rinse with cold mineral or purified water and add 1 tablespoon of cider vinegar for dark hair or

1 tablespoon of freshly squeezed lemon juice for fair hair.

It is wise to avoid anti-dandruff shampoos because they can have a very drying effect on the scalp, especially if used for long periods.

CHAPTER SIX

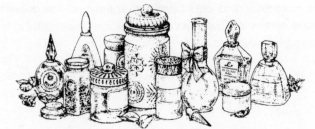

The Female Cycles

Have you ever wondered why women tend to be so capricious? One moment they are assertive and outgoing, the next submissive and introspective. To my mind, these whimsical moods and fancies are largely a consequence of continual fluctuations in the hormones due to her menstrual cycle.

It is only in recent years that we have begun to understand properly the relationship between hormones and emotions. We know that the moodiness and uncertainty of the pubescent years are largely the result of the hormonal upheavals which take place before the menstrual cycle is properly established. But, even after the hormones have apprently 'settled down', a woman goes on experiencing emotional highs and lows, because the different reproductive hormones constantly rise and fall in a rhythmic fashion with each passing menstrual cycle.

This phenomenon has its advantages. For instance, men seem to remain intrigued by the unpredictable and unfathomable nature of women. On the other hand, many women find their hormonal blueprint makes it difficult for them to fit into the rigidity of a nine-to-five occupation, hours that were, after all, established by the men to whom they are well suited. It's not that women are not just as capable as their male counterparts, but they often find it easier to complete tasks at their own pace, and this again is dictated by their hormones.

You will find there are times when you seem to brim with energy and vitality, others when you just want to take things easy and stay at home. If you start making a short note in your diary every day for two or three months concerning how you feel and your attitude to work and the people around you, a pattern is likely to emerge. Being aware of such changes can be a tremendous asset, for it allows you to let your hormones work *for* you rather than the other way around.

In this chapter, I shall look at the ways in which aromatherapy relates to the menstrual cycle, many peculiarly female problems, pregnancy, childbirth and the menopause, and how essential oils can help to treat the kinds of problems that arise when the female hormones fail to harmonise.

THE MENSTRUAL CYCLE

The menstrual cycle begins at puberty and continues through a woman's life until menopause, unless of course it is interrupted by pregnancy and lactation. This cycle involves the participation of several different hormones, which interact in a complex fashion to bring about the maturation of ova within the woman's reproductive organs, the ovaries. Presiding over this process is a region of the brain called the hypothalamus.

In young women puberty usually takes between the age of about ten and fourteen, although it can begin outside this time span. During this time, the hypothalamus starts to send signals to its second-in-command, the pituitary gland, often referred to as the master gland, for it appears to orchestrate the activities of all the other hormone-producing glands in the body. The pituitary responds by releasing what are known as 'gonadotrophic hormones' into the bloodstream. The first of these is a follicle stimulating hormone (FSH). It travels to the ovaries where it instigates the maturation of an ovum within its own little capsule, biologically termed a graafian follicle. As the ovum develops, the follicle starts to produce the ovarian hormone oestrogen. By the time the ovum is fully matured, the pituitary has released another of its secretions, called luteinizing hormone. When this hormone reaches the ovaries it triggers the release of the ovum from the graafian follicle in a process known as ovulation.

The empty follicle, now referred to as the corpus luteum, starts to produce the hormone progesterone. Meanwhile, the mature ovum, which is now highly receptive to the presence of any male sperm, begins its journey along a channel, known as the fallopian tube, towards the uterus. If no sperm are available, and the ovum is not fertilised, it is lost from the body. At the same time, the lining of the uterus (or endometrium) which has been proliferating since the time of ovulation, begins to break down and is shed as blood in a process known as menstruation. On average, this menstrual flow usually lasts from four to five days, although it may be as few as three or as many as seven days long.

The whole cycle usually takes about twenty-eight days, although it is not abnormal to find it can be up to seven days longer or shorter. The first day marks the beginning of menstruation with ovulation taking place around the fourteenth day, but again this varies from one individual to another.

The Menstrual Cycle and the Sense of Smell

The notion that different odoriferious molecules can affect the menstrual cycle is a fascinating one, and it is also highly plausible, for the nerve cells of the olfactory organ are directly linked to the limbic region of the brain. In a manner similar to that of the hypothalamus, this organ influences the secretions of the pituitary gland which in turn can affect the quantities of oestrogen and progesterone produced by the ovaries.

Evidence suggesting that a woman's menstrual cycle can be affected by the pheromones aired by people around her comes from studies carried out on women living in institutions who have little contact with men. It has been observed, for example, that girls in boarding schools develop a menstrual synchronism which is disrupted when a member of the opposite sex appears on the scene. Interestingly, in the presence of men, women also appear to have shorter menstrual cycles, (less than twenty-eight days) than they do if they are apart from men. This suggests that the woman's body is trying to make the most of this opportunity by stepping up the frequency of ovulation, which increases the chances of conception occurring.

To reinforce this possibility, the quality of a woman's pheromones, which are found on her skin, in her hair, and in her bodily secretions such as urine, sweat, faeces and vaginal secretions, also change throughout her menstrual cycle. They become progressively sweeter from the first day of her period, reaching a peak at ovulation. At this time, they are at their most tantalising and can cause men to become quite aroused and excited if they are detected.

This natural attractant wears off as menstruation approaches and during the menstrual flow women secrete yet another kind of pheromone called trimethylamine. This substance, similar in its chemistry to musk, is also produced by bitches on heat, which explains why dogs, rather embarrassingly, often become excited by the smell of menstruating women.

Not only do the pheromones a woman produces change throughout her menstrual cycle, but so does the acuity of her sense of smell. Up until quite recently, the fact that women exhibited acute sensitivity to certain odours was put down to the fact that they didn't smoke and drink as much as men, as both these things affect the sense of smell. But as far back as 1890, a German scientist called Dr Wilhelm Fliess noted a possible link between the sense of smell and the menstrual cycle. He observed that during menstruation the capillaries in the nose became dilated and sometimes even bled a little.

But it was not until 1952 that a French scientist, Dr Le Magnen, established a definite link between sexuality and olfaction. One of his studies involved experiments with a substance called exaltolide which can be extracted from angelica. He tested the reaction of men, women and children to this musky-smelling substance chemically akin to a pheromone found in the glandular secretions of male civet, wild deer and beavers – and found that adult women who were at the ovulation stage of their menstrual cycle were the only ones responsive to this odour.

Le Magnen's work was revolutionary in its suggestion that women's responsiveness to musky odours – chemically very similar in nature to the male hormone testosterone – was related to their menstrual cycles. It is also interesting to discover that women are a hundred times more receptive to such smells around ovulation than during any other period of their menstrual cycles.

I have often found that the essential oil of angelica is very effective for treating women who have lost the sharpness of their sense of smell. This may happen following a bout of illness such as a cold or flu, or around menopause when women often complain of tiredness. I also discovered that in Malaysia the women frequently take angelica as a fertility remedy, while the men use ginseng.

Since Le Magnen's pioneering work, much more evidence has emerged which suggests that the sense of smell is influenced by the reproductive hormones. We now know that women on the pill do not respond to the musky odours so similar to male pheromones, presumably because the hormones within the pill prevent ovulation from taking place. Neither do women who are going through the first few months of pregnancy, possibly because there is no longer any need to be attracted to the opposite sex. Women who have had their ovaries surgically removed or who are going through the menopause and have very low levels of oestrogen and progesterone in their bodies seem to lose the acuity of their olfactory sense too.

Being aware of the alterations in your sense of smell can be very useful to you. I discovered that my own sense of smell was at its peak twelve to sixteen days after the first day of menstruation, and I liked to work in the laboratory at this time, for I was inspired to make new preparations and perfumes. Work was much harder around the time of my periods, and often proved fruitless as the products were not up to scratch. Making such observations helped me to economise on my time, and spare me the frustration of wasted effort.

Why not make a note in your diary every day concerning the way you respond to the smells of foods, perfumes and so forth, and see if you notice any pattern relating to your menstrual cycle emerging? Such observations could also be harnessed in creating a new method of natural contraception, which involves using your nose to pinpoint the time of ovulation.

Other changes that take place throughout the menstrual cycle can act as useful guides too. For example, women will find that their moods and attitudes are affected by their hormones. They may discover they are most extrovert and confident at the time of ovulation. They feel attractive, find it easier to make decisions, and generally have great energy and drive at this time. Such feelings usually start to wear off as the time of their period approaches.

Before menstruation, women tend to become muddle-headed and clumsier. They are unlikely to be able to deal with stress as well as they normally do, and may feel rather irritable and desperate as a consequence. They will also be more inclined to spend time on their own. Primitive tribeswomen actually hide away so they can be by themselves when menstruating. In the West, many women are so difficult to live with around this time that their male companions might well wish they would hide themselves away too!

Most women are unlikely to notice the changes in the quality of their own pheromones during the menstrual cycle, although their male partners might. However, they can be aware of the changes in the nature of their vaginal secretions, which tend to be more copious around ovulation time, and dry up almost completely just before menstruation.

All these things could be used to find a period of time when it is unlikely for conception to take place following intercourse. For on a twenty-eight-day cycle, we know that ovulation will occur some time between the twelfth and sixteenth day after the first day of your last period. Bearing in mind that sperm can live for up to three days, the unsafe period spans from days nine to nineteen. This leaves about a fortnight when it would be safe to have intercourse, namely the four to five days following the end of menstruation and the nine days before the next period is due.

Naturally, the desire to have intercourse will be strongest around the time of ovulation when all the bodily systems are geared towards it, and this is when a reliable but temporary form of contraception such as the diaphragm, should be used together with a spermicide if you do not wish to become pregnant.

Of course, not everyone's periods are regular and you

have to use the knowledge of your own body to work out a timing system which will be effective for you. Women who have been taking the contraceptive pill should also be aware that a few months will have to pass before their natural menstrual cycles are properly re-established.

I have mentioned natural contraception because I feel that the contraceptive pill falls very short of supplying the perfect method. Once hailed as the women's sexual liberator, back in the 1960s when it first appeared on the scene, the pill is now considered a health hazard to many women. Apart from causing unpleasant side-effects such as migraine headaches, depression, irritability, weight gain and oedema, studies now show that pill-taking can be linked to cancer of the breast and cervix. Many women suffer circulatory disturbances when taking the pill and it is thought that these might increase their chances of suffering a heart attack. Indeed, it is also hypothesised that the high levels of hormones circulating in the blood as a consequence of being on the pill may affect the sexual tendencies of a child born to a mother taking it from a very early age.

To my mind there is plenty of scope, and a great demand, for a more sophisticated means of contraception based on observations of natural bodily functions. It is time for the scientists to put their heads together and come up with the perfect – that is, a much more natural – form of contraception.

MENSTRUAL AND OTHER PROBLEMS

Most women suffer upsets in their menstrual cycles at some time during their life, and these can usually be traced back to some kind of hormonal imbalance. The sort of symptoms that accompany such upsets are diverse and are likely to be of an emotional as well as physical nature. Sometimes women are given prescriptions for drugs such as diuretics or tranquillisers to relieve the symptoms, and perhaps even hormones in the form of the contraceptive pill or implants in an attempt to redress the imbalance.

The trouble with such remedies is that they fail to get to the heart of the problem. Because the hypothalamus, pituitary gland and ovaries are all involved in the menstrual cycle, it is likely that the imbalance comes from one of them being either under- or overactive. And one of the reasons why stress is such a problem for women today is because it affects the hypothalamus, which in turn transmits its disturbances to the ovaries and other glands, so disrupting the finely tuned balance. The sex glands not only play a role as organs of reproduction, but also relate to feelings of general well-being in the body: when they are not functioning properly, feelings of tiredness and listlessness set in.

Essential oils provide a safe and effective means of treating menstrual disturbances because they appear to stimulate the endocrine glands and work towards normalising the hormone secretions. Dr Jean Valnet, a leading French expert on aromatherapy, referred to certain essential oils as being menagogues – they act to normalise and promote the menstrual cycle – and such essences are valerian, artemisia, basil, cinnamon, cumin, lavender, melissa, mint, clary sage and thyme. A possible explanation for their influence is that certain essences closely resemble the female hormones. Cypress, for example, is believed to have a chemical structure akin to one of the ovarian hormones, whilst hops also contain a substance very similar to oestrogen.

In this section I have outlined some of the most common problems associated with the menstrual cycle, and how to treat them gently and safely with essential oils.

Amenorrhoea

This is the absence of menstruation. During puberty, it is

not abnormal for a girl to experience one or two periods, and then miss them for the next six or even twelve months. In later life, however, amenorrhoea is often a sign that something is amiss as far as health is concerned.

Women suffering from anorexia nervosa often stop menstruating. This is because the body requires many nutrients, such as vitamins A, E, F and the B complex, together with minerals (in particular zinc), plus sufficient calories before it can synthesise the hormones involved in the menstrual cycle. A shock or severe emotional stress can also interfere with the cycle, as it affects the hypothalamus which in turn may stop the production of female hormones. It is also likely that illnesses such as tuberculosis and diabetes will disrupt the normal pattern of menstruation too.

Women who frequently miss periods or who have only brief and very scanty ones can benefit by drinking tisanes made from sage (which is highly oestrogenic) mixed with camomile as often as possible, as well as using sage in their cooking.

Another treatment is to make an oil to add to the bath, or to rub into the tummy and back.

1 eggcup of soya oil
2 drops of tarragon
2 drops of sage
2 drops of juniper
2 drops of camomile

Mix these together and use in whichever way you like.

Dysmenorrhoea

Many women experience a degree of discomfort when their menstrual flow begins. This takes the form of headaches, backache and abdominal cramps that can sometimes be so painful that it is often best to lie down in a darkened room and rest.

It is often a good idea to seek out foods rich in calcium and magnesium before a period is due to begin, as they are needed for muscle relaxation. Foods rich in the B complex vitamins, especially B6, are also helpful. Liver provides this, as well as the mineral iron lost during menstruation, so it is a good natural way of replenishing the body's supply. Some vegetables – spinach, for example – also contain worthwhile quantities of iron.

To ease the pains, drink plenty of herbal teas such as caraway and the same ones prescribed (following) for premenstrual tension. Avoid taking baths that are too hot.

Make an oil to massage into your tummy and lower back whenever you feel the need.

2 drops of camomile essence
5 drops of parsley
1 drop of tarragon
1 eggcup of soya oil

Pre-Menstrual Tension

Around half the women who come to my clinic complain that, a week before their period is due to begin, they suffer from a number of diverse physical and emotional upsets. Many of their symptoms stem from excessive water retention which makes the tissues of the hands, ankles and face swell, cause the stomach to become distended, the breasts to feel very tender, and the legs to feel exceptionally heavy. Sometimes women gain seven or more pounds in weight in the form of fluid around this time, become constipated, and often complain of migraine-like headaches, which can be the result of excess fluid creating pressure on the capillaries in the head.

Many women also find that their skin may erupt in blemishes and that it generally becomes oilier, as does their hair, before their period. Some complain that their circulation becomes sluggish around this time, and others find they develop the symptoms of a mild cold.

Invariably these physical disturbances are accompanied by mood swings as well. Many find they feel irritable, frustrated, anxious, miserable, and prone to fits of temper and tears. They also talk of being foggy-headed and clumsier than usual. Many of these emotional upsets are linked to low blood sugar, a problem that seems to be hormonally related and leaves women with strong cravings for something sweet and satisfying in between meals.

Insomnia is another pre-menstrual symptom, for women who are tense or depressed often find it very difficult to drop off, and invariably just as difficult to wake up too.

The precise hormonal disturbances that bring about such symptoms still remain rather a mystery, but scientists now tend to believe the problem lies with an imbalance between the hormones oestrogen and progesterone. It is possible that during the week before a period, oestrogen levels in the blood remain unusually high, whilst progesterone falls too low, creating an imbalance between the two. These hormones seem to work antagonistically, so whereas oestrogen encourages fluid retention, progesterone combats it.

The secretion of both these ovarian hormones is under the control of the pituitary gland, so a deficiency here could certainly upset the balance. The pituitary in turn is greatly influenced by the hypothalamus, in the brain, and this controlling centre also responds to stress and other psychological disturbances. This helps to explain why premenstrual tension can vary in severity from month to month, and why sufficient relaxation is very important around this time if you wish to keep the symptoms under control.

There are a number of different steps to take which can

lessen and sometimes totally alleviate the symptoms of pre-menstrual tension. Sufferers should eat small, regular meals, choosing foods rich in the B complex vitamins, particularly vitamin B6 (found in whole grains, nuts, meats such as liver, and fish like cod, tuna and sardines, sprouting seeds, avocados and soya beans), whilst avoiding refined carbohydrates such as white flour, sugar and things made with them like biscuits, cakes, and pastries, as well as fried, fatty foods.

Some women who come to see me eat very little for fear of putting on extra weight at this time, and live off coffee to flush out the excess water, and tranquillisers to soothe their nerves, which are in a state of agitation from the coffee. As a consequence their symptoms often become even worse. Eating regularly is essential, for it keeps the blood sugar at a constant level and staves off cravings.

The mineral magnesium is also very useful, as it has a tranquillising action, and foods rich in this nutrient such as almonds, walnuts, raisins, oatmeal and fish should be included in your pre-menstrual diet. Women should not resort to diuretics to banish their excess fluid related weight, as they bring about the loss of potassium and other important minerals in the urine, and this results in feelings of even greater depression and fatigue.

Taking plenty of not-too-strenuous exercise such as walking, swimming and yoga is also helpful as it releases tension which otherwise builds up inside, and so are periods of quiet relaxation.

Aromatherapy treatments include drinking plenty of herb teas instead of stimulants such as tea, coffee, and alcohol. Useful infusions can be made from parsley, mint, calendula (marigold) flowers, and camomile mixed with orange flowers. This last named herb tea has a soporific action and is very good for those suffering from insomnia. Always boil the teas for 2 minutes and infuse for 5 minutes.

When cooking season your food with sage, basil and thyme, as they make food easier to digest. Indigestion is often a problem before menstruation and sufferers should always try to eat early in the evening to prevent this phenomenon which is yet another cause of insomnia.

Take two warm baths a day, and add 6 drops of essential oil of parsley and 2 drops of neroli, or 4 drops of pine, 2 drops of parsley and 3 drops of neroli. Afterwards go and lie down on your bed for 10 minutes in a darkened room, placing a pillow under your knees.

Make an oil by adding 4 drops of parsley and 3 drops of neroli to 1 eggcup of soya oil. Massage this mixture into your abdomen, lower back and the back of your neck.

Cystitis

Cystitis is a condition characterised by an inflammation of the bladder and it can be extremely painful and debilitating. Bacteria co-exist in large numbers in a healthy bladder, but if something disrupts the balance, an infection can occur which gives rise to this inflammation.

Women on the pill are more prone to cystitis than most, because the hormones in it can alter the bacterial flora in the urethra as well as the vagina. Illnesses such as bronchitis, a bad cold accompanied by sinusitis, and even a severe chill may provoke a urinary infection too. On the other hand, the cystitis may be initiated by irritants such as kidney stones.

Certain smells such as that of fresh paint can also cause irritation and I know of many cases of women whose cystitis attacks have coincided with the decoration of their house.

Even frequent sex stimulates the proliferation of bacteria in the urethra in some women. A simple remedy for this is to drink plenty of tepid water after intercourse, as this cleans out the bladder. It is also worth remembering that women who take little exercise are also more prone to suffering from cystitis, for their weak muscles encourage the retention of urine within the bladder.

The best treatment for cystitis is to keep warm and make a herb tea by boiling the wispy hairs found on corn on the cob for 10 minutes. Drink five to six large glasses of this infusion per day – and eat the sweet corn at meal times.

An infusion of cherry stalks also makes a good diuretic for cystitis sufferers. Mix about 3 pinches of stalks in 500 ml (a scant pint) of water and boil for 2 minutes, then infuse for 5 minutes. Or boil 450 g (1 lb) of cherries plus their stalks in 1 litre (2 pints) of water and drink the syrup first thing in the morning.

To a warm bath, add 5 drops of sandalwood, pine, juniper or parsley oils.

You could also make a massage oil by adding 6 drops of any of the essences above to 1 eggcup of soya oil. Massage into the tummy, lower back and sacral region, then apply hot and cold compresses alternately.

Cellulite

Although cellulite is invariably referred to as a physiological disorder, it may be some comfort to know that most women suffer from it some time or another. To my knowledge, women have always had cellulite, but it only became a problem when they started wearing bikinis and scantily clad young models with waif-like figures began adorning the pages of glossy magazines.

Cellulite is brought on by a hormonal change which encourages the body tissues to retain water, invariably characterised by high levels of oestrogen. When the fat cells become interspersed with this water, the skin takes on an orange peel appearance when squeezed between the fingers, and often feels uneven and bumpy too. Cellulite usually appears on the thighs, buttocks, hips, sometimes the stomach and the upper arms, and even the back of the neck too.

Because cellulite is hormonally related, mild forms of it can come and go, so women may find they have it before periods and that it disappears when their period begins. Pregnant women also seem to have cellulite as this is another time of hormonal upheaval, as do women going through their menopause.

The severity of the condition and whether it becomes a permanent fixture or not depends a good deal on lifestyle. Because stress affects the hormonal balance, nervousness, tension, frustration, shock, anger and so forth can all bring on a cellulite condition, and it is important to relax if you don't want it to stay around. Bad circulation also predisposes women to cellulite, so if your hands and feet feel cold and your skin bruises easily, you will have to take extra care. Hormonal imbalances are often responsible for circulation problems, but so is bad posture, in particular flat feet. It can also go hand in hand with an underactive thyroid gland. A sluggish circulation can be speeded up by taking regular exercise (swimming and walking are perfect), and by following a warm bath (never hot) with a cold shower.

Certain foods also encourage a cellulite condition for they provoke fluid retention. These are salty and smoked foods (cured hams, etc.), sugar, refined carbohydrates such as white flour, and things made from it. Women with allergies to certain foods such as milk, which causes the tissues to swell, will also be prone to cellulite, as will women who have a poorly functioning liver.

Strangely enough, diuretic drinks such as tea, coffee, and alcohol – especially spirits – actually worsen the condition, so it is wise to stay away from them.

TREATMENT
Before a bath, rub your body with a loofah to activate the circulation. Add the following essences to the bath water (which should never be too hot).

2 drops of cypress
2 drops of lavender
2 drops of lemon (good for the circulation)

Finish with a cold shower, and then rub the following oil into the affected areas.

3 drops of cypress
3 drops of sage
3 drops of lemon
1 eggcup of soya oil

Drink plenty of sage and vervain teas. Take kelp tablets to supply the iodine needed for the thyroid gland or, if they tend to keep you awake at night, dissolve a few in your bath water.

Look for foods containing plenty of vitamin C (citrus fruits, blackcurrants and cherries), for it is a mild diuretic. In nature it is found together with bioflavinoids such as rutin (found in the flesh and skin of citrus fruits) which helps to strengthen the blood vessels and promote a healthy circulation.

For a herb tea rich in both these nutrients, boil the skin of a lemon in 500 ml (a scant pint) of water and leave overnight before adding the juice of the lemon. Drink this first thing in the morning, diluted with a little spring water if you wish. Finally, try and drink several glasses of mineral water each day as this in itself is an effective antidote to fluid retention.

Leucorrhoea

This is an inflammation of the vagina often caused by the proliferation of unwanted bacteria or even a kind of fungus which gives rise to a thick discharge which is white or yellow in colour. It often occurs if women have been taking a course of antibiotics. Women who are most susceptible are those using the contraceptive pill, those who are pregnant, or those suffering from the metabolic disorder diabetes.

To prevent leucorrhoea, a good diet is essential, one which is particularly rich in foods containing vitamin A and the B complex vitamins. Avoid wearing underwear made from synthetic fibres such as nylon or polyester, as well as tightly fitting jeans.

TREATMENT
Add to your bath 2 drops of juniper or 2 drops of lavender. You can also use just 1 drop of either of these essences when using a bidet or douching.

PREGNANCY AND CHILDBIRTH

The nine months of pregnancy can be the happiest of your whole life. This is partly because, from the time of puberty, a woman's body has been awaiting the occurrence of this very phenomenon, so no wonder it brings such a tremendous feeling of fulfilment. You will be carrying something born of love, and it is a wonderful feeling to experience it growing within you. For me, every day of my pregnancy was exciting, and I felt exceedingly contented the whole time.

During pregnancy it is very important that you are healthy and fit, for your physical and emotional state will have great bearing on your child's development. It is particularly essential that you take special care of yourself during early pregnancy for, from the time of conception through the first eight weeks, the foetus is developing at a phenomenal rate.

The foetal cells need a plentiful supply of all the essential vitamins, minerals, amino acids, fatty acids and so on if they are to grow and reproduce, so it is very important to eat well at this time. Pollen is an excellent supplement to take, for it contains all the nutrients essential to health, so try taking ¼–½ a teaspoon every day. Also give up stimulants such as tea, coffee and alcohol, replacing them with camomile, sage and rosehip tea with honey if you wish. Drugs should be avoided in pregnancy where possible.

Studies also point to the fact that breathing in noxious fumes that contain chemicals or toxic minerals such as lead can also be highly damaging to the developing child and may even cause miscarriage. Remember, poisonous things do pass from the mother to the foetus, so it is important to protect your baby from anything that could be dangerous at this vunerable stage.

Pregnancy is characterised by an upsurge in the production of oestrogen and progesterone. Such hormonal changes can bring about certain other changes. You may experience cravings for certain foods and smells and find others make you feel nauseous. Other discomforts may include oedema (swelling), circulation problems, sleeplessness and in the late stages, nervousness.

Essential oils provide an excellent means of treating such things and will generally enhance your feeling of well-being too. Because they reach the bloodstream, the essences will also pass to the baby who benefits from them as well. However, I must point out that certain odoriferous substances can be abortants, so it is never a good idea to play around with them. The ones I have prescribed are known to be safe, and the recipes specially devised so they are present in balanced proportions.

Oedema

During pregnancy fluid can be retained by the tissues. It affects most women because it is a normal physiological adjustment which provides extra protection for the foetus. You should never try to combat it with strong diuretic tablets, as these not only flush out the water but take away essential minerals such as potassium and magnesium and this could be damaging to the baby.

If your tissues swell excessively you should step up your intake of vitamin C, which has a mild diuretic action. Some essential oils contain substantial amounts of vitamin C – the citrus ones, orange, mandarin, and lemon, for instance. Make a massage oil by adding 1 drop each of petitgrain, orange and rose to 4–5 teaspoons of almond oil. You can also add the pure essences to your bath.

Circulatory Problems

Varicose veins may develop if you do not take care. This is because the expanding womb constricts the blood flow to the limbs, and the extra weight you are carrying makes it harder for the blood to return from the extremities to the heart.

Look for foods rich in vitamin E to help the circulation, as well as those containing vitamin C. Bioflavinoids are also important, because they strengthen the blood vessels and are present in the skins of citrus fruits as well as in pollen granules.

Another good way of helping the blood flow is to place a pillow under your mattress at the end of the bed, so you are lying at a slight angle. Alternatively, place a couple of blocks of wood under the bottom of the bed to raise it slightly off the ground.

Make a massage oil by adding 3 drops of cypress, 2 drops each of lavender and lemon to 1 eggcup of soya oil. Massage into the legs especially. You could also add the pure essences to your bath.

Women may also suffer from piles (haemorrhoids) as a result of bad circulation in which case they should try to sit in a basin of very cold water and massage with the oil recommended on page 56.

Nervousness

It is important to stay calm and relaxed during your pregnancy, for nervous problems such as tension and anxiety will not be very good for the child.

The mineral magnesium is essential for good nerves, which is why it is often referred to as nature's tranquilliser. Almonds are a good source of this mineral, so nibble around twelve to sixteen every day, and add them chopped to fruit salad or muesli. They also contain phosphorus, linoleic acid (one of the essential fatty acids), vitamin A and the B complex vitamins (also needed for healthy nerves).

Many essential oils have a sedative action on the nervous system and are very helpful for massaging and inhaling during pregnancy. Make a nerve tonic by adding 2 drops of neroli and 2 drops of melissa to 4–5 teaspoons of soya oil. Rub into your chest and tummy, and you could also add the pure essences (2 drops of each) to your bath.

Insomnia

From about the sixth month of pregnancy onwards it may become quite difficult to sleep as your baby starts getting active. To ensure a good night's sleep it is a good idea to select foods such as lettuce, which has a soporific effect, as well as oranges and mandarins, and do not go to bed after a heavy meal.

Before retiring to bed, drink an infusion made by boiling a pinch of lavender and a pinch of bigaradier (orange flowers), in 500 ml (a scant pint) of water for 2 minutes. Leave to steep for 5 minutes and take 2 cups, sweetened with a little honey. Or place a little cup of water with 1 drop of lavender and 1 drop of neroli near a radiator, so that it perfumes your bedroom and helps you to drop off.

Preparing for Childbirth

When your baby is ready to be born, the hypothalamus tells

the pituitary gland to release a substance called oxytocin, which stimulates the contraction of the uterine muscle. When I was in Malaysia, I discovered that the women use a lot of nutmeg in their cooking during pregnancy because it strengthens and tones the muscles and primes them for contraction.

Two to three weeks before the baby is due, massage your tummy with the following.

3 drops of nutmeg
2 drops of sage
1 drop of neroli
4–5 teaspoons of almond oil

Also sprinkle grated nutmeg on your vegetables as this will help their digestion too, and add it to the milk you are undoubtedly drinking.

During Childbirth

Essential oils can be very helpful during labour, as they can ease breathing difficulties and promote relaxation.

For breathing, rub an oil made from 1 drop each of pine, eucalyptus, and neroli, and 3 teaspoons of almond oil into your chest. For relaxation, add 1 drop of neroli and 1 drop of lavender to a bowl of warm water and leave it beside your bed, so that the vapours disperse in the air.

During the early part of pregnancy, a gentle back massage using the oil you have chosen will help you to relax, and aid the circulation, as well as reducing oedema. But it is not advised to massage the back after the third month. In advanced pregnancy, a leg massage is tremendously beneficial, and it is also a good idea to get someone to rub the oils into the soles of your feet.

Breast-feeding

After childbirth a substance called prolactin is released by the pituitary gland, which stimulates the glands in the breasts to produce milk. The constituents of this milk are derived from the blood flowing through the glands, so the baby continues to receive all the nutrients he needs in a well balanced form from his mother after he is born.

A very special kind of milk is produced during the first few days after childbirth, called colostrum, and it is very important that the baby receives this milk if he is to be strong and healthy. This is because colostrum contains antibodies which lend protection against foreign substances until baby is capable of making his own. This early protection fills what is called 'the immunity gap', and this is why babies fed on breast milk are far more resistant to infections than those fed by bottle. Another reason why breast milk is best is because babies often have allergies to cow's milk which manifest themselves as colic, eczema, vomiting, diarrhoea and anaemia.

Breast-feeding should be a joy to the mother, helping to intensify the bond between her and her baby. But many women are put off by the thought that their breasts may sag. On the contrary, breast-feeding helps them regain their shape. During the last nine months of pregnancy the hormones oestrogen and progesterone have been priming the glands for milk production, and when a mother breast-feeds the suckling action tones up the muscles which gives her breasts support. So it is only when their function is neglected that they suffer.

Some women complain of sore, cracked nipples which make breast-feeding a painful experience. To prevent this happening, massage a mixture of almond oil and lemon juice into the nipples all through pregnancy.

After childbirth, massage the whole breast with an oil made from 4 drops of rose, 2 drops of lemon, and 2 teaspoons of almond oil, which will encourage them to regain their firmness.

To stimulate a good flow of milk, add fennel, carrots and lentils to your food as often as you can, and also eat plenty of parsley – chopped in salads, with steamed vegetables, or as a juice (if you have an extractor), mixed with fruit juices. Drink a herb tea made by boiling a few hops in water for 2 minutes. Leave to infuse for about 5 minutes and drink a few cups as required.

Aromatherapy for the Baby

It is quite a shock for a baby to leave his secure little world inside the womb and to arrive in a strange new one, so he will need comfort and reassurance through touch and pleasant aromas. To his first bath add just 1 drop of lavender or neroli. Because his sense of smell is quite sophisticated at this early age, you will notice that he will probably be surprisingly responsive.

Never wash him with a harsh detergent soap. If his face is a little greasy, some witch-hazel mixed with purified or distilled water will do nicely instead.

After drying baby, give him a gentle massage using light stroking movements with an oil made from 1 drop of neroli, 1 drop of lavender and 1 eggcup of almond oil.

INSOMNIA
If a baby of over 3–4 months has difficulty sleeping, prepare an infusion of orange flowers by adding 1 pinch to 500 ml (a scant pint) of water, boil for 2 minutes and leave to infuse for 5 minutes. Sweeten with honey and give this drink to him in between feeds.

COLIC
Sometimes the reason why a baby cries and cries and seems uncomfortable is because he has colic. For a baby of 3 months and over, a good remedy is to boil some sliced carrots together with a piece of fennel for 45 minutes. Strain, add a teaspoon of honey and give this to him when

he cries. You could replace with a camomile tea made with 2 herbs, and 1 teaspoon honey.

Fill his bedroom with soothing aromatic vapours by soaking a piece of cotton wool in water containing a few drops of pine and orange essential oils, or lavender and orange. Squeeze out the excess water and leave the pad on or near the radiator.

MENOPAUSE

Most women living in the western world view menopause with great apprehension, for they see it as marking the beginning of old age and the end of their good looks. The idea that beauty lies only in possessing an elegant silhouette and a youthful complexion is one that is unfortunately perpetuated by many glossy magazines and serves to enhance the fear of menopause.

But the truth is that menopause is simply the end of the menstrual cycle, just as puberty signifies its onset. It happens because the ovaries gradually cease to respond to the stimulation of the gonadotrophic hormones produced by the pituitary gland. This usually starts to occur between the ages of forty-two and fifty, although it can happen much earlier if a person is suffering from malnutrition, emotional stress, or poor health brought on by illness. As a consequence, the menstrual cycle becomes irregular and eventually stops altogether.

Several different physical and emotional upheavals are linked to the diminished production of oestrogen and progesterone. Many women suffer from hot flushes, excessive sweating, spells of dizziness, weakness and sometimes a reduced interest in sex: these only take place, however, while the body is acclimatising to the changes, and later on they disappear. In this respect, menopause is similar to puberty, when the upheavals in hormone levels give rise to moodiness, water retention or swelling and occasional dizziness. Women will also find that when they are tired or emotionally distressed these hormone-related symptoms can be exaggerated.

One lady who came to me for treatment was very distressed for she was only thirty-five years old and already beginning her menopause. Her frequent trips to the gynaecologist had proved fruitless, and no wonder, for the hormonal changes were being brought on by her exceptionally erratic way of life. She was a career woman, and during the last ten years, had been travelling consistently between England, California and Asia. On top of this, she had adopted highly irregular eating habits, which contributed to the development of peptic ulcers as well as insomnia.

I suggested that she had a course of relaxing treatments at the practice, and altered her diet. I also formulated some oils for her to use which contained cypress, verbena and rose, along with other essences. They were to be used in the bath, massaged into the skin and taken internally.

Now, she has actually passed through her early menopause, and although she still leads a very active life, the treatments have shown her the importance of relaxing and looking after herself. Now she no longer suffers from the health problems that she did only a few years ago.

Another charming person who had been coming to me for a long time, had begun her menopause quite normally when she was fifty. She was, however, intensely anxious about the idea of getting old, especially as she was married to a man ten years her junior, who was very active. Because she felt she was losing her looks, she shied away from sex, and this problem was intensified by the fact that her husband told her he would soon have to start looking for a younger woman. At the time she was also suffering from indigestion, constipation, cystitis, insomnia and cellulite, which she felt were linked to her menopause.

Searching for clues as to why this should be, I discovered that she ate nothing all day, drinking tea and coffee to keep her going, because she waited to have dinner with her husband. Because they usually ate between nine and ten o'clock at night, she was not digesting her food properly, and this was the main cause of her gastric problems and insomnia, not her hormones at all.

I prescribed sassafras and eucalyptus for her cystitis, sage to correct the hormonal imbalance and ease nervous tension as well as thyme to improve her bad circulation and combat her insomnia.

Treatment

For anyone going through menopause, I would recommend sage and nettle teas, for they are rich in substances akin to the female hormones, whilst sage is also good for hot flushes. Thyme is very beneficial for nervous problems and can take the place of tea and coffee as a stimulant without creating the difficulties they do.

For those suffering from insomnia, an infusion of passiflora (passion-fruit flowers) should help them get a good night's sleep.

Make a massage oil to rub on the tummy and into the back of the neck.

3 drops of thyme
2 drops of rosemary
3 drops of basil
3 drops of cypress
1 eggcup of soya oil

To your bath add either 3 drops of basil and 3 drops of cypress; 3 drops of thyme and 3 drops of rosemary; or 3 drops of rosemary and 3 drops of basil.

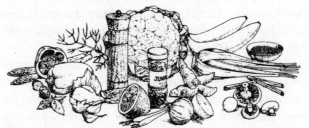

CHAPTER SEVEN

Aromatherapy in the Kitchen

In recent years, there has been a growing awareness of the nutritional value of fresh, 'whole' foods, but sadly, the importance of their *aroma* has remained neglected. This is a pity, because aroma plays a number of essential roles in the choice, preparation and cooking of food. In France and Italy, before any purchase is made, the discerning customer will often touch and always *smell* the foods on sale. This is because food aromas give subtle clues as to their quality, indicating whether, for example, the meat is fresh or the melons are ripe.

Unfortunately, most of us have neglected our sense of smell, and consequently have also lost the power to judge foods by their aroma. It is easy, of course, to tell the difference between fresh and sour milk, but how many could guess the flavour of melons from their fragrance?

We now rely too heavily on the appearance of foods, usually judging the freshness and quality by colour and plumpness and juiciness, and food manufacturers have learnt to exploit this. It is not unusual to find packaged meats containing a red colouring to make them look fresher, and chickens which have been injected with substances called polyphosphates before they are killed to make them look succulent. You will also find many so-called 'fresh foods' are sealed in polythene wrappers which prevent any odoriferous molecules from escaping, and will probably have difficulty in persuading any shopkeeper to let you smell his wares!

Aroma plays an important role in the preparation of food, as well as its selection, as it primes the body to receive nourishment. When you squeeze fresh oranges first thing in the morning, you are not only extracting a juice rich in vitamin C, you are also inhaling a delicious aroma which wakes up the digestive processes. (It may even evoke memories of sundrenched holidays in Tunisia or southern Italy for some.) Of course, if you buy the tinned or cartoned varieties, the olfactory organ is not stimulated in the same way, which is why it is so worthwhile spending a few extra minutes on preparing fresh fruits instead.

Delicious aromas should similarly pour forth when food is cooking to encourage a good appetite. For, when odoriferous molecules are detected by the olfactory organ, nerve stimuli are sent to the brain, which in turn triggers the secretion of saliva and gastric juices. An appealing aroma also enhances the pleasure received from eating a meal. Again, this is due to the fact that the part of the brain associated with smell (the primitive limbic region) also controls feelings of contentment. Such an association probably arose from the need to make those processes emotionally rewarding that were necessary for our survival.

For this reason, it is a good idea to prepare food for anorexics and depressives – who have lost the incentive to nourish themselves – with many herbs and spices. Such condiments are particularly evocative to the olfactory organ, because they are rich in aromatic essential oils which are released from foods when they are chopped, squeezed or crushed, and heated.

The essential oils in foods also encourage good digestion within the body, the value of which is, again, frequently overlooked. No matter how wholesome and vitamin-packed various foods may be, the nutrients sealed in them are of little value if they are not released and assimilated properly. Emotional stresses and strains, fatigue and exhaustion all act to inhibit the flow of digestive juices which means that food will only be partially broken down, which is why anxious and nervous people frequently suffer from indigestion. If semi-digested food particles pass into the bloodstream, they can cause all kinds of discomfort such as headaches, water retention and nausea, so it is well worth incorporating aromatic herbs, fruits, vegetables and spices in your cooking whenever possible.

Essential oils also possess the useful property of being able to fix the minerals present in food, which prevents them from dissolving in the cooking water and being lost down the sink. Nowadays, fruits, vegetables and cereals are grown too fast, due to the use of fertilisers (usually chemical), and they do not have enough time to assimilate all the nutrients they should. Correct cooking is thus vital, as we can ill afford to lose those that are present. Fruits and vegetables should not be cooked at very high temperatures (in pressure cookers, for instance) nor boiled for too long, as such treatment encourages the loss of minerals and destroys vitamin C and some of the B vitamins too.

AROMATIC COOKING IN HISTORY

The essential oils found in herbs, spices, fruits and vegetables have many therapeutic properties, which is why to be a good cook is also to be a good doctor.

Man has been aware of the healing power of certain plants for thousands of years, but it was during the times of the ancient Egyptians that the use of plants as medicines reached a peak of sophistication. Numerous recipes formulated for the treatment of a variety of different illnesses were revealed when the Papyri of Ebers and Edwin Smith were discovered. From these and other sources we learn that the Egyptians took their medicinal cookery very seriously but at the same time took great pleasure in using aromatic substances in this way.

The ancient Egyptians cultivated fields of cucumbers, leeks, wild radishes, and smaller gardens of herbs such as tarragon, parsley and bay, and spices like ginger. To keep epidemics away they added quantities of cinnamon and ginger to their food. Both onion and garlic were often taken to combat physical weakness and tiredness, and because the poor could not afford meat, they would cook an onion instead. Even the lowlier classes knew a good deal about the value of aromatics in cooking. They were aware that certain foods were harder to digest than others, and would skilfully blend them with aromatic herbs and spices. They would add coriander, aniseed and caraway to help the digestion of breads made from rye and millet, a method still used today in some European countries such as Hungary and Germany. When cooking beans, of which they were very fond, they mixed them with onions and thyme to overcome the common problem of flatulence. Wealthier Egyptians would stuff meats and fish with a mixture of wholemeal flour, honey and numerous aromatic herbs.

From texts relating to the ancient Greeks come evidence that Alexander the Great introduced many herbs and spices from Asia and Europe to Greece. Hippocrates, the father of medicine, whose teachings are still referred to today by naturopaths and herbalists, believed in the therapeutic use of aromatic plants through food and cooking. He prescribed onions for people suffering from water retention, chervil for those experiencing melancholy brought on by a liver or stomach malady, rosemary to be added to vegetables to overcome liver and spleen disorders, and mustard for sciatica.

The Greeks would often sit down to twenty-course meals, which I believe would not have been possible without the liberal use of aromatics in their cooking! And Epicurus, the gastronome and philosopher, would insist on the use of at least five aromatic herbs if he were to enjoy a meal.

A distinguished botanist of this time, Theophrastus, was highly respected for his culinary knowledge. He had a special recipe for oysters which were prepared with caraway and pepper to make them easier to digest when eaten in large quantities. Fish would be cooked between leaves of oregano and fennel and served with a sauce seasoned with garlic, onion, tarragon, thyme and pepper. A special ragout was prepared using fennel, parsley and oregano which made meat easier to digest and gave it an appetising aroma too.

Etimus, another culinary expert, was renowned for his lentil stew which he made with caraway seeds and thyme to prevent the iron being lost during cooking. The Greeks also appeared to be fond of a black pudding which was seasoned with garlic, onions, thyme and oregano, and a similar dish is still eaten in regions of France today.

The Romans ate very plain food for 600 years until their conquests took them further afield, and they began to bring back herbs and spices as well as ideas for their use. Many of their dishes were copied from the Greeks, and adapted to suit their own tastes. The Romans held aromatic plants in high esteem. Special recipes using herbs and spices were created to please the emperor of the day and poets would dedicate odes to their favourites. So precious were pepper and cinnamon at that time, as well as salt, that they were used as money.

One of the greatest threats to health at that time was posed by cholera, and to protect themselves the Romans would add rosemary, juniper berries, hyssop and basil to their dishes.

Interestingly, women in those days seemed to be plagued as much by pre-menstrual tension as they are today. To relieve the symptoms, they would add parsley to salads and drink infusions of both the leaves and seeds. This drink was also taken for dysmenorrhoea.

The Romans, like the Greeks, were very fond of their food, and ate such enormous amounts at their banquets that they invariably suffered from halitosis. To sweeten their breath, they would chew bay leaves and caraway seeds. They were particularly skilled in the art of making court-bouillon, a liquor made from wine, herbs and spices such as thyme, rue and chervil, in which they cooked fish. Another popular dish involved leaving a dish of tuna, mackerel, sardines and eel in a marinade of dill, fennel, coriander and thyme in the sun for ten days until the fish had decomposed. They would then bottle this vitamin-rich concoction and eat it with pasta and toasted bread.

In India, strong spices have also been used for centuries in cooking. This practice probably arose from a need to prolong the freshness of meat, which decays at a rapid rate in the hot climate. However, ancient Indian medicine was also based on a use of aromatic foods, and many of the spices used in cooking by other civilisations probably originated from India. The Arabs, who certainly traded at Indian ports many hundreds of years ago, incorporated many spicy aromatics into their cooking as well as their own home-grown oranges and lemons, valued for their subtle perfumes, in baking cakes and other delicacies.

Many traditional French dishes are derived from Roman and Greek culinary practices, and because of the great selection of meats, fish, fruits and vegetables in France they vary from region to region. My father's parents came from the Ardèche and Lozère regions of the South of France, and he was brought up on fine traditional French cookery. He was a well-known poet and writer in France, and would often find inspiration while pondering over a deliciously aromatic dish. He was naturally very appreciative of good food, and I can recall him saying, 'The English are a fine race, but something is missing – a good palate.' Although he visited England occasionally, he would never stay for more than a day because he could not stand the food!

My grandmother, who was a headmistress, grew up in a tiny village where there was no doctor, so whenever possible, ills were treated with therapeutic dishes. I can remember being taken by my grandmother for long walks into the mountains to gather the right herbs for adding to wines and soups. She was especially enthusiastic about wild thyme (called serpolet). If any of us had a cold, she would set about preparing a special meal to treat it. She might take a piece of meat and cook it in water with wild thyme, rosemary, garlic and onion, then make a white sauce with two fresh horseradish roots, which was very strong. Alternatively, she might prepare a soup of potatoes, carrots, celery, celeriac and lots of fresh marjoram. Then for dessert, we might be given rice pudding made with lots of angelica and ginger.

I am still looking forward to the day when you can go into a restaurant and, instead of just being shown the menu, are asked if you have any ailment – a headache, cold or pre-menstrual tension perhaps? – before a delicious aromatic dish is prepared to specification.

GUIDELINES FOR HEALTHY EATING

Good health is not something that can be left to chance: it depends largely on your lifestyle, and to a very great extent on the kind of food you eat. The fresher the food and the less it has been tampered with, the better. This is because all processing techniques – freezing, canning, drying and particularly refining – involve, to a greater or lesser extent, the loss of many vital vitamins and minerals.

In my view such procedures also kill the food. Fresh food
possesses a natural energy, especially fruits and vegetables
which contain active enzymes. Such foods are, if you like,
alive. When foods are subjected to high temperatures or
their structural integrity is demolished, they lose their
energy as well as their aromatic essential oils. In this state
they are of little value to us. Because processed foods usually
end up tasteless. aromaless and colourless, artificial
flavourings and colourings are added, often with preservatives, which have no nutritional value at all. In an attempt
to compensate for the lost vitamins and minerals, manufacturers sometimes add synthetically produced equiva-
lents, but it is unlikely that they are as useful to us as the real
ones.

So when stocking up your larder:

Replace white sugar with honey (unfiltered is best) and
  raw muscavado sugar
Replace white bread with wholemeal varieties
Replace tinned fruits and vegetables with fresh
Replace margarines with cold pressed vegetable oils and
  unsalted butter
Replace instant coffee with freshly ground beans, etc . . .

In other words, try to keep as much as possible to *natural*
ingredients.

When shopping, it is always a good idea to choose foods
that are 'in season', and locally grown. This way it is more
likely that the carrots have just been plucked from the
ground, or the apples have recently been picked from the
tree. Otherwise they may have been in storage for months,
losing vitamins all the while. Exotic fruits and vegetables
may provide interesting variety, but they have probably
been artificially ripened (this is certainly true of bananas),
and they should always be supplemented with home-grown
varieties.

The manner in which food is prepared should also harmonise with the time of year. In winter, when it is cold, greater quantities of body fuel are required (in the form of calories), to generate extra heat and to convert into fat for sealing in the warmth. This is why we can comfortably eat richer foods such as nuts and meats during the winter, but should be drawn towards lighter fare during the warmer months. Could you imagine for instance, eating Christmas cake on a hot summer's day? Vegetables raw in salads or as crudités are ideal for the summer months, but in winter they will be far more appetising steamed with a light coating of butter.

I have found that providing you comply with the laws of nature, and are aware of your body's requirements, any extra pounds that are gained during the winter will be shed naturally when spring arrives. This means you need never bother with boring diets that centre around calorie counting!

The story of eating for good health actually goes beyond simply choosing fresh, wholesome foods. This is because each person has needs for different nutrients which change constantly with the passage of time. For instance, a woman who has passed through her menopause needs fewer calories than a young athletic girl. As women age they also need less protein, and often find meat difficult to digest, especially when eaten in the evening. Many cases of insommnia and indigestion are the outcome of sitting down to an overly rich meal after eight o'clock at night.

Many women fare better if they change their diet to suit their menstrual cycle. Those who retain water pre-menstrually may find eating raw fruits and vegetables in great quantities actually accentuates the problem, and should cook them lightly beforehand (see also Chapter Six).

Periods of stress and emotional upset increase your body's requirements for certain nutrients such as vitamin

C, and the B complex vitamins, so foods containing them should be sought after during such times. An addiction to stimulants such as tea and coffee is often a good indication that you are under too much strain, or that something else is amiss healthwise. (Stimulants are considered as food by some, but are not.) The stimulants themselves are often dismissed as being harmful, and they are taken in excess, but when taken occasionally as a quick pick-me-up, their action can be quite beneficial.

Healthy Eating for the Young

Babies and children have special dietary needs because they grow at such a fast pace and need extra nutrients to build new tissues and strong bones. Unfortunately many women have been brainwashed by manufacturers into thinking that their offspring should eat food that is specially prepared and comes in the form of tinned or dried soups and desserts, crunchy biscuits and cereals with added vitamins, etc. There is a tacit implication that a mother is irresponsible if she does not cater for her child's needs with such foods.

But babies can survive quite happily without such foods, and have done so for hundreds of years. In fact, because many baby foods contain added sugar, salt, colourings and flavourings, they are actually damaging to the young child whose delicate constitution cannot cope with such impurities. No wonder there are so many cases of skin rash and allergy nowadays.

It is infinitely better to give your children the kind of fresh foods you would choose for yourself. When baby is teething, pieces of raw vegetable and fruit such as carrot, cabbage, and apple are ideal as they contain essential oils which help to soothe sore and swollen gums. Make a simple yet nourishing dish by mashing potatoes, and adding other vegetables such as carrots, courgettes, tomatoes, turnips or green beans. Never throw away potato cooking water, but use it for the mashing, mixed with milk, soya milk or fresh cream plus a teaspoon of olive, corn or sunflower oil. Add variety with a little grated cheese such as Cheddar, Gruyère or Parmesan, an egg, some fish like fillet of sole or cod, or perhaps some minced liver. And use other vegetable cooking waters for soups, stocks, sauces, etc.

Always season baby's food with aromatic herbs and spices for he will appreciate their aroma and benefit from their power to help digestion. It is interesting to discover that most children will develop a taste for aromatic foods such as garlic, onion, basil and parsley at a very early age.

After the age of about three, there is absolutely no reason why children should not eat the same food as their parents. When I was a child I always shared meals with the rest of the family which helped to develop my sense of smell and taste, so that even when I was quite young, I was able to discriminate between a good and bad Camembert.

Nowadays children are often given gimmicky foods packed with additives. Because they trust and rely on their parents, children are oblivious to the harm such foods can do (advertising, of course, bears a lot of responsibility for this). Any loving mother who wants her children to grow healthily should always take the time to prepare wholesome meals for them. When baking cakes it is always better to replace white sugar with dried raisins and sultanas, nuts such as almonds and walnuts, honey and bananas. Substitute sweetened puddings with baked apples, fresh fruit salads, rice and semolina cakes. This way a child will not develop cravings for sweets, bought biscuits and cakes, and will actually turn them down when visiting friends.

It is also a good idea to let your child be responsible for making his own foods. Allow him to add his own fruit, nuts and honey to natural yoghurts, which will develop his own skills and tastes. Time spent teaching him the value of food and showing him the ingredients on the packets of convenience and junk foods when shopping is never wasted. And, even if he wants to try something new that he has seen advertised on television, be firm and refuse him. Saying yes is not always the best way of showing your affection and winning his love, and he will certainly thank you for it later on.

KITCHEN UTENSILS

The quality of the utensils used when cooking is as important as the ingredients.

Always avoid using saucepans and baking trays made of aluminium. During cooking aluminium salts can dissolve out (especially when fruits and vegetables are boiled) and mingle with the food. Aluminium interferes with the secretion of digestive juices which gives rise to flatulence, bloating and other unpleasant symptoms.

Avoid cooking in copper too, because it oxidises (characterised by the green colouring often seen on pans) and can be quite harmful. It can also upset the body's stores of zinc, which is highly undesirable if this mineral is already short.

For preference choose enamel or stainless steel saucepans, china dishes, clay pots (ideal for baking bread) and wooden spoons.

KITCHEN ESSENTIALS

Turn your kitchen into a pharmacy by always keeping it well stocked with fruits, vegetables, herbs and spices rich in essential oils, for when used in cooking: they not only produce an appetising aroma and taste, but also add therapeutic properties to your meals. The following listing is only a selection of the many herbs, spices and aromatics which can enhance your cooking – and your health.

Angelica

The name angelica derives from a tenth-century French tale of Archangel Raphael, who revealed the virtues of this aromatic substance to a monk so that he might use it as a weapon against the plague.

Angelica, which grows in northern European countries, Russia and Scandinavia, has a hot flavour and a musky aroma, and is an excellent general tonic. It stimulates the brain and, because it is stomachic, helps digestion and enhances the appetite. Angelica also treats nervous depression and other nerve-related disorders, and promotes good respiration.

Basil

The Greek word for basil is *okimon*, meaning 'quick', because the plant grows so rapidly, but a Byzantine princess, who relished its perfume and beauty, gave it the name *'basilikon'*. In India, the Hindus believed that basil offered protection to the soul in both life and death, so it was frequently used in religious ceremonies to praise the god Vishnu, and at funerals. Rubbing basil all over the body was also thought to help protect those who had nightmares about snakes from the poisonous venom. In Egypt the aromatic fumes of basil were offered to the gods, and the essences mixed with myrrh and incense were used in embalming.

Its therapeutic properties are rather controversial, because there are so many different varieties of basil. Generally, it is a good diuretic, and a nerve and stomach fortifier. It gives relief from difficult periods, dyspepsia, insomnia and migraine. Women suffering from swollen breasts when pregnant may find a compress of rose water and infused basil helpful.

When dried, basil can be smoked instead of tobacco, and

is good for asthmatics. Basil goes well in salads, and in some parts of France and Italy the leaves are served on their own. It also enhances the flavour of soups and ragouts.

Bay Leaf

Bay belongs to the same plant family as cinnamon and camphor. The essential oils in its leaves and berries are good for treating dyspepsia, flatulence, loss of appetite (particularly in anorexics), those with scanty periods, bronchitis or tonsillitis. It makes an effective remedy for flu and any other viral infection accompanied by fever, as it promotes sweating.

For flu, boil 20 g (about ¾ oz) of leaves with some berries in 500 ml (a scant pint) of water and drink 2–3 cups a day. If you have an infection, boil some bay leaves and inhale the fumes.

For dyspepsia, add 2 bay leaves and the peel of half an orange (not sprayed with chemicals) to 200 ml (7 fl. oz) of boiling water. Infuse for 15 minutes. This is good for flu as well.

Add bay leaves to marinades made with white wine, shallots, garlic, pepper and cloves and leave the meat in this for 3–4 hours prior to cooking.

Caraway

Caraway seeds have an aroma similar to that of fennel, being hot and spicy. The ancient Egyptians were very fond of mixing caraway into breads to make them more digestible, as well as soups and onion dishes.

Caraway has anti-spasmodic (relieves muscle spasm), stomachic and carminative properties, and is very good for dyspepsia. Those suffering from indigestion can benefit from drinking an infusion of caraway seeds, ½ teaspoon per 300 ml (½ pint) cup of boiling water.

In France, caraway is often mixed with cheese, and pork

is cooked with it to help the digestion. Those who find wholemeal bread difficult to digest should mix some caraway seeds, fennel and aniseed with butter and spread it with this mix.

Chervil

Chervil was known to the Greeks as *poederos*, which means 'children of love', and its present rather less romantic name was chosen later by a botanist. Today, fifteen different kinds of chervil can be found growing in Europe. It is very good for treating all kinds of bladder disorders such as kidney stones and cystitis. It is a potent diuretic and helps to correct bad circulation and troubles associated with it like haemorrhoids, vein problems and cellulite. It also benefits people with high blood pressure.

A soup made with potatoes and chervil is helpful for anyone with kidney stones, and when celery is added, which maximises the effects of chervil, it is very beneficial for cystitis sufferers too. Anyone who suffers badly from water retention before their period will find relief in drinking a few cups of herb tea made by infusing 20 g (about ¾ oz) of lettuce and 10 g (just under ½ oz) of chervil in 500 ml (a scant pint) of water.

Add the seeds mixed with fresh leaves to salads and omelettes, sprinkle over soups and stews, and stir into fresh home-made mayonnaise.

Cinnamon

In ancient Chinese medicine, cinnamon was looked upon as a panacea, and around 2700 BC no prescription was considered complete without it. Cinnamon is one of the oldest spices known and was used not only by the Chinese, but also by the Romans, Greeks and ancient Egyptians, who always added it to their wines and meals.

It actually originates from Malaysia and Sri Lanka, and

has a distinctive hot, peppery aroma and taste. It is a good remedy for flu (see Chapter Four) and also helps to treat fatigue and depression.

Clove

Cloves were discovered by the Arabs when their travels took them to the Molucca Islands off the east coast of Africa. They then spread to Malaysia, Sri Lanka, and the Seychelles. In China it was considered respectful to chew cloves before meeting the emperor for this purified the breath.

Clove is one of the most effective antiseptics known and is good for treating all kinds of infections such as flu and colds. It benefits people suffering from rheumatism and helps to ease the pains of childbirth, so women in labour should take wine steeped with cloves at frequent intervals.

Coriander

Coriander originated from the East and was later introduced to North Africa, Egypt and Greece. Today a good deal of coriander is grown in France and Morocco, and it is valued both for its leaves and seeds.

The ancient Egyptians believed that a drink made by steeping coriander seeds in wine had the power to bring happiness, and another reference cites it as promoting a good night's sleep. In India, coriander is still used a good deal in preparing curries for it halts the putrefaction of meat.

Coriander also fortifies the stomach and sweetens the breath. It gives relief from headaches and sometimes depression, providing it is used in small quantities. It restores a good appetite, so it is useful in the treatment of anorexia, and helps the digestion of difficult foods such as cabbage. Coriander seeds can be added to vinegar, and they transform mushrooms into a particular delicacy.

Fennel

Fennel is a very decorative and aromatic plant which has long been regarded as a potent diuretic, and can be taken for this purpose in wine, liquor or vinegar. Its other therapeutic properties include being a stomachic, stimulant, galactagogue (stimulating the secretion of milk after childbirth), and a mild laxative. It also provides a useful remedy for cystitis, a weak bladder and asthma, and when taken in Bordeaux wine is good for easing a cough.

An infusion of 1 tablespoon fennel herb to 500 ml (a scant pint) of water can be applied to the eyes to reduce itching and inflammation brought on by an infection. Fennel seeds go well with cucumber and vinegar, and can also be mixed with cheese and sprinkled over steamed vegetables. A delicious white sauce can be made for serving with asparagus by adding finely chopped fennel herbs and lots of fresh parsley.

Garlic

Like onion, garlic is strongly antibiotic. It not only keeps colds and viral infections away, but drives them out too, so speeding recovery from illness. A good source of iodine, garlic is highly recommended for anyone with an underactive thyroid gland, who suffers from poor circulation, or has a weight problem. My grandmother would use garlic cloves as suppositories when we had a cough or cold as children. It also benefits anyone with high blood pressure or a rheumatic condition.

Raw garlic is best, so add it crushed to steamed vegetables. Also place a clove in 150 ml (¼ pint) of cold pressed olive oil and use the flavoured oil in salad dressings as well as cooking. Those who object to garlic's potent aroma on their breath should chew some fresh parsley or a few coffee beans after a meal.

Ginger

This hot spicy root comes from India and Malaysia, and its name comes from the Sanskrit *zingiber*. It has always been renowned for its digestive properties and is actually good for any gastric upset such as nervous dyspepsia and travel sickness. It also has a reputation for being an effective aphrodisiac, especially for those older people, and is more tonic than pepper. Those suffering from rheumatism can benefit by drinking an infusion made from 1 root of ginger, a sprig of marjoram and a sprig of rosemary boiled in 500 ml (a scant pint) of water. If too bitter, reduce the quantity of herbs, especially marjoram.

In cooking, ginger complements the flavour of many jams and marmalades, and improves that of plain or vanilla ice cream. It should always be added to winter dishes as it provides warmth.

Juniper Berries

Both berries and leaves have a strong aromatic fragrance and in ancient times were burned in religious ceremonies to purify the air and ward off the plague. The berries are tonic, stomachic, diuretic and good blood cleansers. They can benefit people suffering from arthritis, rheumatism and liver infections like hepatitis.

When ground, they made a good substitute for pepper, and can be added to sauerkraut together with caraway seeds. They also go well with game and are often added to wines or liqueurs like Chartreuse.

Lemon

Always keep a good store of fresh lemons, for they are not only highly nutritious, being rich in vitamin C, but also provide a handy first-aid kit. If you cut yourself, always apply lemon juice, even though it stings, for it sterilises the wound. Rub it into mosquito and flea bites to reduce the inflammation, and massage it into your children's feet if they suffer from chilblains in the winter. Rub your hands with lemon juice before handling meat and fish to cleanse and disinfect them, and afterwards to remove any odours that may have impregnated the skin.

Lemons possess antiseptic properties, and when taken internally keep coughs and colds away. One of the best remedies for sore throats and mouth ulcers is to gargle with lemon juice.

If children have worms make a purgative drink by boiling the skins of 3 lemons in 500 ml (a scant pint) of water. Leave to stand overnight, add the juice of 1 lemon, and give to them first thing every morning.

Lemons purify the blood and promote good circulation. Anyone suffering from cellulite, blemished skin, vein problems or rheumatism will benefit from drinking lemon juice in water or tea, and using it in their cooking.

Marjoram and Oregano

These herbs are one and the same, but whereas marjoram is cultivated, oregano grows wild in the mountains. Marjoram was considered sacred by the ancient Egyptians who offered it to the god Osiris for his pleasure, and similarly in India, the people believed that it would please the gods Shiva and Vishnu. In Greek mythology a legend tells how the goddess Aphrodite applied marjoram to heal the wounds suffered by her son, Aeneas.

Both are stomachic, expectorant and sedative, and are helpful in the treatment of insomnia, migraine, dysmenorrhoea, and diarrhoea. In cooking, they enhance the flavour of meat and help the assimilation of minerals from it. They are excellent in marinades, especially for pork. For each 450 g (1 lb) of meat, use 400 ml (a scant ¾ pint) of white wine, 4 pinches of marjoram or oregano, and the grated peel of 1 orange.

Add them to stews, minced meat, stuffed tomatoes, peas, beans and salads. When mixed with cabbage, Brussels sprouts and turnips, they help digestion and prevent flatulence, which can sometimes be a problem with these vegetables. They go particularly well with overpowering cheeses as they tone down their aroma and make them easier to digest.

Mint

Mint is one of the best known of all the herbs and grows in abundance in Britain as well as in the mountains of Provence and around Paris in France. Its name derives from *mente*, a Latin word meaning 'thought', because it stimulates the brain.

The Greeks believed it capable of preventing menstruation. It is also thought to be good for the voice, so perhaps singers could benefit from taking it, and it helps to heal ulcers, excites the appetite, gives relief from insomnia and dyspepsia, fortifies the nerves, and is an excellent expectorant (relieving mucus). A tisane or tea of mint – 75 g (2 oz) of mint leaves in 1 litre (2 pints) of water – should be taken for coughs and colds; for bad catarrh, it is even better with eucalyptus added.

Onion

Onion possesses potent antibacterial properties, and everyone can benefit from eating it daily for it helps keep colds and infections at bay. It has a sound reputation for correcting glandular imbalances, and is often recommended for people with a weight problem.

The presence of the mineral sulphur gives onion excellent skin conditioning properties, whilst silica promotes strong bones and a good blood supply to all body tissues. Onion is also an effective blood cleanser and helps to correct poor lymphatic drainage, which is so often responsible for oedema and puffiness.

Raw onion is best because when cooked it loses many therapeutic properties. Those who find it difficult to digest should add some, very finely chopped, to a little olive oil and leave for at least an hour and a half, so the essential oils can disperse before using the oil to dress salads. Once your tolerance starts to improve, you can add minced raw onion to soups and steamed vegetables.

Pepper

Pepper has always been regarded as a very precious spice. Its name actually comes from the Sanskrit word *pippali*, although the Greeks called it *pepperi*. It was considered to be a good aphrodisiac and the French, who adore it, still use a lot of whole peppercorns in cooking dishes such as steak *au poivre*. Mixed with ginger, hyssop and thyme, it is even more effective, apparently, at stimulating a sexual appetite. It also activates the secretion of saliva, gastric and pancreatic juices, and ensures good digestion, especially of fat. Pepper is valued for its anti-putrefactive properties, which is another reason why it is good with meat; and because it helps to tone the muscles, it is very good for athletes and anyone wishing to firm up.

Parsley

The name parsley comes from the Greek word *petroselinuon*, which means 'herb-dissolving stones'. It shares many therapeutic properties with chervil, with regards to the bladder and kidneys. Parsley is also helpful in treating liver problems such as biliousness and jaundice, as well as menstrual difficulties like dysmenorrhoea, amenorrhoea and pre-menstrual water retention. An infusion of pure extracted parsley juice can be useful in treating eye problems, and the juice can also be helpful when applied to bee stings and bruises. A drink to treat tonsillitis can be made by boiling 50 g (2 oz) of parsley in 500 ml (a scant pint) of water and adding honey to taste.

When cooking fish, make a sauce for it with lemon and parsley, for this herb helps the digestion of protein. Its delicate aroma also reinforces the flavour of white meat, and when added to omelettes, benefits the action of the liver.

Parsley is a rich source of vitamin C, so use it the whole year round sprinkled into soups, salads, and dishes made with beans and lentils.

Rosemary

This is perhaps the best known and used aromatic herb. The Greeks and Romans, who believed it symbolised love and death, used it in religious ceremonies and feasts. It was also favoured by the ancient Egyptians, and traces of rosemary were found when the tombs of certain pharaohs were excavated.

The term rosemary actually comes from the Latin *rosmarinus*, meaning 'rose of the sea', for it can be found growing wild along the coast in most Mediterranean countries.

The herb is strongly antiseptic and is also a stimulant, cholagogue (benefiting the liver), and diuretic. For rheumatic conditions add 50 g (2 oz) of rosemary to a litre (2 pints) of dry white wine and leave to stand for four weeks. When ready drink a little warmed wine with honey. Taken this way it is also good for women suffering from water retention.

If a red wine does not appear to have a very good bouquet, add a sprig of rosemary to it and leave overnight to enhance its aroma. Because of its antibacterial properties, rosemary goes well with poultry, rabbit, lamb, in fact any meat which may putrefy, and it also helps the digestion of fat. In Italy it is frequently added to rice dishes, while in France rosemary is used to perfume hams.

Sage

Since antiquity sage has been regarded as a sacred herb. Its name derives from the Latin verb *salvere*, to save, and it appears to benefit any ailment.

The ancient Egyptians gave it to women who were unable to bear children, and also valued it as a remedy for plague. According to the memoirs of Saint-Simon, a writer well acquainted with the goings-on at the French court, Louis XIV took an infusion of sage every night before going to bed, and it was to this that he attributed his long and fruitful life. The Chinese still value it so highly that they will give 4.5 kg (10 lb) of their tea for just 450 g (1 lb) of sage leaves.

Sage is renowned for helping to promote and normalise menstruation. It can also be used for treating rheumatic conditions, catarrhal discharge, haemorrhage, and excessive sweating, and is recommended for convalescents.

It is an excellent seasoning for meat dishes such as lamb and pork, and goes very well with onion and garlic. For a herb tea good for almost anything, infuse 2 tablespoons of sage leaves in a litre (2 pints) of water.

Salt

Salt is not an aromatic herb or spice, but it is an excellent condiment. The Greek writer Plutarch believed it to be the finest of all condiments, and it stimulates the secretion of saliva which is the first stage of digestion.

Always buy sea salt in its most natural form and use in moderation as it encourages the tissues to retain water. Those suffering from oedema, high blood pressure or obesity would be wise to replace it with herbs.

Savory

The Greeks believed savory possessed strong aphrodisiac properties, and its virtues were sung by Virgil. In France during the seventeenth and eighteenth centuries it also had a reputation for stimulating a sexual appetite, and was thought to promote or normalise menstruation and fortify the stomach too.

The name savory (*sarriette* in French) is derived from the Latin *satura*, meaning 'herb for stews'. In cooking it should be added to dishes of beans, peas, and lentils, for it helps the assimilation of their vitamins and minerals, and aids their digestion: one of the best remedies for post-bean flatulence! It is also delicious mixed with cheeses, together with sage, and gives a subtle perfume.

An effective aphrodisiac can be prepared by infusing savory with sage and a few peppercorns, and drinking them when the need arises. (It contains natural hormones which dynamise the sexual glands.) A fine aromatic dressing for salads may be made by steeping savory, together with a few juniper berries, chopped onion, and shallots in wine vinegar and leaving for two weeks.

Tarragon

This herb, which originates from South Russia, has a very strong, aromatic fragrance similar to anise, and was much favoured by the maharajahs of India who took it as a tisane. It is stimulant, stomachic, diuretic and a mild laxative, and provides a helpful treatment for dysmenorrhoea and intestinal parasites.

Tarragon is excellent in sauces like Béarnaise for red meats and chicken, and can be mixed into salads too. It makes a useful alternative to salt for people suffering from heart problems or obesity. An infusion of 2 tablespoons of chopped tarragon in 1 litre (2 pints) of water acts as an effective diuretic.

Thyme

Thyme grows wild in the South of France and other Mediterranean countries. Its use can be traced back to the ancient Egyptians who incorporated the essential oils of thyme into embalming fluids. The Greeks, who named it *thumos*, meaning 'smell', were known to drink an infusion of thyme at the end of a banquet. It is a tonic, stimulant, pectoral (good for the chest), and helps treat asthma, flu, coughs, fever, nervousness, as well as aches and pains.

If afflicted by a bout of gastritis, drink an infusion made by boiling 2 tablespoons of thyme with a little mint in 1 litre (2 pints) of water, throughout the day. When applied externally, infused thyme can also reduce the swelling associated with rheumatism and oedema.

Thyme fixes the iron in meat and makes it easier to digest too. For both fish and meat, make a marinade by adding 1 tablespoon of thyme, ½ tablespoon of savory, 4 cloves of garlic, 4 shallots, 2 bay leaves, 4 cloves and 10 black peppercorns to a litre (2 pints) of white wine. This herb also helps the digestion of potatoes, beans and lentils, and makes a welcome addition to many soups and stews.

Vanilla

When Cortez travelled to Mexico in the sixteenth century, he discovered vanilla was being used by the Aztecs to flavour a hot chocolate drink which they used to take after meals as a stimulant.

Vanilla possesses many therapeutic properties, for it is a tonic, antiseptic, digestive and stimulant. In Paris during the eighteenth century, vanilla was added to chocolate in varying concentrations, and was sold in chemists' shops as stomachics and pectorals (good for the chest and bronchitis). A hundred years later, vanilla was also being prescribed in France for young girls suffering from melancholy.

Because vanilla is so helpful in the digestion of rich foods, it is a good idea to use it in dessert recipes such as ice cream, soufflé and even fresh fruit salad.

AROMATIC RECIPES

Although a number of very good cookery books have been written, I always find the recipes within them very difficult to use. This is because I cannot follow the reasoning behind the mixing together of so many diverse ingredients. So little thought appears to have been given to the compatibility of different foods, which is why elaborate dishes are frequently hard to digest and leave you feeling overburdened and uncomfortable.

Good food should certainly be a pleasure to eat, but it must also be kept simple and light. Although you should be satisfied after eating, you should also feel clear-headed, stimulated and energetic.

Always try to use the very best ingredients – cold pressed virgin olive oil, the finest and freshest vegetables, free-range chickens, etc. – as these, although expensive, will be the tastiest and most healthful. The following selection of recipes not only taste good but, with the use of aromatics, also *do* you good!

Onion Soup

Serves 4

450 g (1 lb) onions	Salt and pepper
A little olive oil	2 pieces wholemeal bread
1 tablespoon wholemeal flour	100 g (4 oz) grated cheese (Cheddar, Gruyère or
1 litre (2 pints) water	Emmenthal)
1 bay leaf	1 teaspoon grated nutmeg
1 sprig of thyme	

Slice the onions and fry in olive oil until golden brown. Add the wholemeal flour and slowly stir in the water. Add bay leaf, thyme and a little seasoning and leave to simmer for 20–30 minutes.

Meanwhile toast the bread and cut into cubes. Place in bowls and pour the soup over. Scatter with grated cheese and a sprinkling of nutmeg, and place under the grill to brown before serving.

As a child, I can remember coming home from weddings and similar occasions where rich food had been served. Our maid would greet us with this onion soup, for it is a perfect antidote to over-indulgence, due to its cleansing properties. It is an ideal dish for the winter and it is also a soothing remedy for colds and flu. It will benefit anyone suffering from skin troubles, insomnia, cellulite, obesity, or circulatory problems.

Sage and Garlic Soup

Serves 4–6

6 large cloves garlic
1.5 litres (3 pints) water
100 g (4 oz) vermicelli, millet or whole semolina
Salt and pepper

4–5 sage leaves
2 tablespoons olive oil
50 g (2 oz) Parmesan cheese, grated

Place the whole cloves of garlic into a saucepan with the water, and bring to the boil. Simmer for 20–25 minutes, then add the vermicelli, millet or semolina, and season with salt and pepper. Continue simmering for 10 minutes, then add the sage leaves.

Remove the garlic cloves and crush them to a paste with the olive oil. Remove the soup from the heat and stir in the garlic paste. Serve hot with a generous helping of cheese.

This is a good soup for people suffering from arthritis,

rheumatic troubles and pre-menstrual tension. It would also be good during pregnancy, because of sage's calming effect, and might help the digestion during the first few months of pregnancy, when nausea could be a problem.

Carrots Vichy

Serves 2–3

1½ tablespoons olive oil
1 onion, thinly sliced
6 large carrots, thinly sliced
1 cardamom clove
1 bay leaf

1 sprig fresh thyme (or pinch dried)
Sea salt
150 ml (¼ pint) water
1 clove garlic
Parsley and/or single cream

Heat the oil in a saucepan and gently fry the onion and carrot slices with the cardamom until golden brown. Add the bay leaf, thyme, sea salt and water. Cook very, very slowly for 15–20 minutes (depending on the quality of the carrots). Half-way through cooking time add the crushed garlic.

When cooked, turn into a serving dish and sprinkle with freshly chopped parsley, and you could even pour in a little single cream to make a delicious sauce.

This vegetable dish is rich in vitamin A, and is ideal for the winter months as it increases resistance to infections. It is especially good for people with liver problems (without the cream), diarrhoea, constipation, anaemia and rheumatism.

Spicy Lentils

Serves 4

700 g (1½ lb) lentils (soaked overnight and boiled until soft), plus their cooking water

1 tablespoon coriander seeds
½ teaspoon caraway seeds
½ teaspoon mustard

1 onion, finely chopped
1 clove garlic, finely
    chopped
5 tablespoons olive oil

powder
½ teaspoon freshly ground
    black pepper
Thyme and sage
Salt

Fry the onion and garlic lightly in the olive oil, then add all the other aromatic herbs and spices. Finally stir in the lentils and their cooking water. Add a little salt to taste. Simmer for 12–15 minutes. Serve with fresh parsley, chervil or tarragon sprinkled on top.

This dish makes a good winter meal, accompanied by meat (especially ham) or potatoes. It is also good in the summer, served cold with new potatoes, or mixed into salads. If to be served without meat – for there is a lot of protein in lentils – add more onions like the ancient Egyptians would have done!

This is a very nutritious dish, packed with vitamins and minerals. It is good for children, pregnant women, old people, athletes and academics suffering from mental fatigue!

Oregano Mushrooms

Serves 2 as a main dish, 3–4 as a starter

700 g (1½ lb) mushrooms
Juice of 1 lemon
1 clove garlic, crushed

Oregano and/or coriander
    seeds
Olive oil
Fresh parsley and chervil

Slice the mushrooms finely, pour the lemon juice over to prevent them turning brown, and put in a frying pan. Cook them just as they are, and afterwards add the garlic, oregano, and olive oil (perhaps some sliced kidneys if desired).

Serve on hot toast, sprinkled with fresh chopped parsley

or chervil.

Mushrooms are a good source of protein, so can happily be eaten by themselves without meat (although these are particularly delicious with kidneys). The use of oregano or coriander is important, as they help the digestion of a substance called chitin, found in the cell walls of fungi, which most of us find difficult to digest.

Garlic Baked Potatoes

1 medium potato per person	*Plenty of rosemary*
	Olive oil
1 clove garlic per person	*Sea salt*

Scrub and cut the potatoes lengthwise into three. Spread in a dish and cover with sliced garlic, rosemary, a brushing of olive oil and a sprinkling of sea salt. Place in a pre-heated oven at 350°F/180°C/Gas 4 and bake for about 15 minutes. Reduce the heat to 300°F/150°C/Gas 2, and bake for a further 15–20 minutes until golden brown and cooked all the way through. Serve with salad.

This is good for everybody, in the winter months especially, as the garlic and rosemary keep colds and flu away, and both are good for the digestion. It is an excellent way of giving children garlic without making them feel they're taking a medicine!

Garlic Bread from Tuscany

1 piece of wholemeal bread per person	*A few cloves of garlic*
	Cold pressed olive oil

Place the bread in a pre-heated oven (350°F/180°C/Gas 4) for 5–10 minutes until toasted. While still hot rub each piece with a clove of garlic (with some ripe tomato as well, if you like). The garlic will sink into and soften the toast.

When serving, pour over the olive oil, as much as you like, and accompany with raw vegetable salad.

This dish is very good for children who always seem to be unwell, for it builds up their resistance to illness. It's also a more palatable way of taking garlic than swallowing a garlic perle every day, so can benefit everyone.

Basil and Tomato Sauce

900 g (2 lb) tomatoes
2 medium onions, sliced
  finely
Olive oil
3 garlic cloves

Bay leaf, coriander seeds,
  and lots of fresh basil
  (10–15 leaves)
300 ml (½ pint) water

Cut the tomatoes into cubes and fry them with the onions in olive oil, adding all the herbs. Simmer gently for 25 minutes with the water.

You can add grated Parmesan, Gruyère or Cheddar cheese if you like. Keep it in the fridge and use in place of bought tomato sauce. It makes a perfect sauce for pasta, rice or cod steak.

This is a good dish for people with pre-menstrual tension, or nervous headaches and migraine. The acidity of the tomatoes with the basil helps the digestion of the carbo-hydrate in pasta, which can cause flatulence. The Italians obviously appreciate this: who's ever seen a pizza without tomato?

Natural Mayonnaise

Makes about 150 ml (¼ pint)
1 clove garlic
1 teaspoon mustard

1 dessertspoon cider
  vinegar or lemon juice

1 egg yolk   *150 ml (¼ pint) olive oil*
                               Herbs or spices of choice

Crush the garlic clove and put in a bowl along with the mustard, egg yolk, and a little of the vinegar or lemon juice. Beat together thoroughly. Add the olive oil very slowly – one drop at a time to begin with – beating vigorously all the while. When the mayonnaise has thickened (when about half the oil has been added), add the rest of the vinegar or lemon juice. Carry on adding the oil, and beating until the mayonnaise is the desired consistency. Add a little paprika, basil, parsley or tarragon depending on the dish with which it will be served. Paprika is best for white meat; tarragon and basil are good with raw vegetables, for instance.

The clove of garlic will help your mayonnaise to be firm. If you are suffering from an ailment, add a herb or spice which will benefit you, referring to the listing at the beginning of this chapter.

Cottage Cheese

1 litre (2 pints) milk (with   *4–5 garlic cloves*
   the cream)   *Chives or basil*
Juice of 1 lemon   *Paprika*

Bring the milk to the boil slowly, then add the lemon juice, stirring continuously. When the milk has curdled, pour it into a colander, lined with a piece of muslin, sitting over a pan or bowl. Cover with a plate and leave until all the liquid has drained away. The next day, add crushed garlic and finely chopped chives or basil to the curd, and sprinkle with a little paprika.

This is a good summer dish and goes very well with a fresh, green salad, or spread on wholemeal bread. The cheese is pure protein, with lots of calcium, so you don't need any meat with its fat. Different herbs add different therapeutic properties, so choose those to suit your needs as well as your palate.

Meat and Offal

Nowadays, cattle, sheep, pigs and chicken are often given antibiotics to keep infections at bay, and hormones to make them put on weight, all of which we absorb when we eat the meat. For this reason it is best to eat meat in small quantities, and not too often.

Always cook meat with aromatic plants, for the flesh starts decaying the moment the animal is killed, and may contain harmful bacterial toxins. Chicken, for example, is often responsible for food poisoning. The decaying process can be slowed down by herbs and spices because they check bacterial growth, and they help to neutralise any harmful substances which may be present too.

Always remove any visible fat before cooking meat, because it is not only bad for you, but it is also here that the hormones will be most concentrated.

Meat is also digested better when cooked or served with aromatic substances. This is why traditionally lamb is served with mint sauce, and pork is served with apple sauce containing cloves. In France pork is actually cooked with rosemary and garlic, but it will be followed by an apple dessert or Calvados (apple brandy). Cheaper cuts of meat are best casseroled with vegetables, and should always have lots of herbs too.

Because liver and kidneys are organs of elimination, they will contain toxins which need to be drawn out; there are two ways of doing this. Either soak thin slices in milk and thyme for one hour at most, and then dry thoroughly before cooking with lots of aromatics such as sage, oregano, bay leaves and juniper berries. Or, for kidneys only, slice very thinly and flambé in alcohol (which counteracts the toxins and makes them easier to digest).

In France kidneys are fried very quickly in olive oil, garlic, onions and herbs, then simmered for about 15 minutes. Liver and heart can be treated in the same way: sage goes particularly well with liver, as it helps fix the iron in the liver, and helps digestion in general.

Fillet of Beef

Good quality meat requires little cooking. For each 450 g (1 lb), make two holes in the top and bottom and insert a clove of garlic, a few leaves of thyme and some pepper into each. Seal the meat with a coating of olive oil. Never sprinkle with salt, as this draws the juices out of the meat, and these contain many essential minerals. Never turn the meat with a fork once it's started cooking either, as this has the same effect.

Pre-heat the oven to 500°F/250°C/Gas 9, then reduce to 400°F/200°C/Gas 6 before putting in the meat. Bake for 25 minutes per 450 g (1 lb). A well-cooked piece of meat should be very crispy on the outside, and graduate through pale pink to bright red in the centre.

Fillet is the least fatty meat, so means fewer potential cholesterol problems, but when being cooked it needs some help to prevent it drying out – thus the healthier vegetable-oil coating. The garlic and thyme inside the meat helps digestion of the protein, and they fix the minerals, especially iron.

Tarragon Chicken

Serves 4

1 small chicken, about
  700 g (1½ lb)
Whole fresh tarragon
  leaves

Juice of 1 lemon
Salt and pepper

Make small incisions all over the skin of the chicken, and slip the tarragon leaves under it so that the whole chicken is covered. Also squeeze in the lemon juice, season with the salt and pepper, and put the prepared chicken into a pre-heated oven (450°F/230°C/Gas 8). Cook for about 35–45 minutes until golden brown and keep pouring away the fat as it drops into the pan.

Chicken should be eaten much more as it is the least fattening meat. But it still contains some fat, and this particular cooking method – inserting a herb between the skin and the flesh – ensures the melting and draining of the fat off the bird. The dish is good for those who can't normally digest the fat in chicken, and the tarragon is especially good for pre-menstrual tension.

Rice Cake

175 g (6 oz) rice	*Grated peel of 1½ lemons*
1 litre (2 pints) milk	*2 teaspoons freshly grated*
2 sticks cinnamon	*ginger*
4 eggs, beaten	*165 g (5½ oz) brown sugar*
30 g (just over 1 oz) butter	*or 100 g (4 oz) honey*
or fresh cream	*Juice of ½ lemon*

Wash the rice, place in a saucepan, cover with water and boil for 2–3 minutes. Remove from the heat, strain and rinse under cold water. Meanwhile bring the milk to the boil in another saucepan with the cinnamon. Add the rice and cook slowly for 30 minutes until the rice has absorbed all the milk. Blend in the eggs, butter or cream, lemon peel and ginger. (You can remove the cinnamon if you like, but the taste is more concentrated if you leave it in throughout the cooking.)

Make a caramel with the brown sugar or honey and lemon juice by cooking slowly together until brown. Mix with the rice and pour into an oven-proof dish. Cook slowly in a pre-heated oven (400°F/200°C/Gas 6) for 30 minutes.

Eat when it has cooled slightly, or chill in the fridge and cut into slices like a cake when very cold.

This was a recipe of my grandmother's, who made it for us when we were children. It is a good packed lunch ingredient for children as it is full of protein. It's also a good winter cake as the ginger is effective for coughs and colds.

Apple Cinnamon

Serves 2, 3 or 6 (depending on appetite!)

550 ml (1 pint) milk	*Fresh lemon juice*
75 g (3 oz) brown sugar	*Powdered cinnamon to*
6 slices wholemeal bread	*taste*
1 egg, separated	*A few raisins*
700 g (1½ lb) eating apples,	*4 teaspoons honey*
thinly sliced	

Sweeten the milk with sugar, then soak the bread in it until soft. Mix into a paste and add the egg yolk. Whisk the egg white until stiff, and then blend it into the mixture. Add the apples, lemon juice and cinnamon. Place in a dish and top with raisins and honey. Place in a pre-heated oven (350–400°F/180–200°C/Gas 4–6) and bake for 30 minutes.

This is a good dish for everyone, especially children. In the apple season, it makes an interesting change from crumbles or pies, being a cross between apple crumble and bread and butter pudding. It is particularly good after a pork or lamb dish, as the apple and cinnamon help the digestion of the fats in those meats.

Crème Caramel

Serves 4
*4 tablespoons honey or
  brown sugar*

1 vanilla pod, split	Sauce
550 ml (1 pint) milk	50 g (2 oz) rose petals
3 eggs, beaten	250 ml (½ pint) water
	5–6 tablespoons honey or brown sugar

Add the honey and vanilla pod to the milk and heat until just about to boil, then take the saucepan off the heat. Pour in the eggs and blend together, then turn into an oven-proof dish. Place the dish in a pan of water – a *bain-marie* – and put into a pre-heated oven (300°F/150°C/Gas 2) and cook for about 45 minutes until the caramel has fully set.

For the sauce, boil the rose petals in the water for 2 minutes and leave to infuse for 15 minutes. Strain and add the honey or sugar, then put the syrup back into the saucepan and heat slowly for another 15 minutes. Pour this liquid over the caramel and leave in the fridge to chill for at least 6 hours, otherwise you will not taste the rose sauce.

This dessert is excellent for people suffering from sore throats, tonsillitis, or who have had teeth removed; rose acts on the mucus as well, and helps alleviate coughs. It is a nourishing dish for children and is also good for women suffering from pre-menstrual tension (a good salad and a small helping of this would be a good meal around this time).

AROMATIC WINES AND LIQUEURS

A fine wine is the ideal accompaniment to a carefully prepared meal, for it helps the digestion and generally enhances the joy of eating.

The reason why white wine traditionally accompanies white meats like fish and poultry, and why clarets and Burgundies go with beef and lamb dishes is mainly due to the compatability of tastes. However, dry white wines are best with fish because they make it easier to digest.

Two glasses of good wine drunk with a meal should be ample, and any more is unnecessary. It is not advisable to take wine between meals as it is absorbed into the bloodstream very quickly and literally goes to the head. Always opt for the higher quality wines which come from small vineyards, because many of the mass-produced wines contain chemicals, and it is often these that bring on the symptoms of a hangover – dry mouth and headache – rather than the wine itself. When I discovered that such wines have been known to dissolve the metal containers in which they are stored, it explained why they can have such a toxic effect on the human body.

Wine also acts as a good carrier for the essential oils of aromatic substances, and wines perfumed with herbs and spices have been drunk for thousands of years. To the Greeks such wines could stimulate the appetite for food and sex, and bring about a state of relaxation and euphoria. They also possessed various therapeutic properties, so rose would calm and beautify, violet would help people with congestion, aniseed would treat dyspepsia, and coriander would ease menstrual difficulties.

The recipe for one famous Greek wine has been in existence for over 2,000 years. It contains fifty-four different aromatic substances such as ginger, cinnamon and aniseed, but the exact recipe is a closely guarded secret.

The ancient Egyptians also drank a variety of aromatic wines, one of these being sage, which was often given to women who were infertile. The Romans took ginger wine for its aphrodisiac properties, prescribed thyme for anorexia and dyspepsia, and myrtle wine for those with weak stomachs.

Here are a few simple recipes you can try for yourself.

Aromatic Vermouth

1 litre (2 pints) white wine
1 stick cinnamon or ½ tsp
  powdered
Grated peel of 1½ medium
  oranges (well washed)

6 cloves
½ teaspoon coriander
  seeds
¼ teaspoon grated nutmeg
½ teaspoon aniseed

Add everything to the wine, and leave to stand for four weeks. This is an excellent aperitif to stimulate the release of gastric juices.

After-Dinner Liqueur

2 litres (4 pints) vodka
  or rum
500 g (2 lb, 2 oz) brown
  sugar

Grated peel of 4 fresh
  lemons
6 vanilla pods, split
2 slices of angelica root

Add everything to the spirit, and leave to stand for three to four weeks. You can also use this liqueur to flavour cakes, especially the rice cake on page 145. This drink will help the digestion of the meal.

Vanilla Wine

1 litre (2 pints) Malaga or
  Madeira wine

3 vanilla pods, split

Leave the vanilla in the wine for three to five weeks. A small glass drunk after meals is good for people with a cough or who smoke.

Angelica Wine

1 litre (2 pints) Malaga
  wine

50 g (2 oz) grated or sliced
  angelica root
1 small ginseng root

Add the roots to the wine and leave to infuse for six weeks. This is an excellent tonic.

Cinnamon Wine

1 litre (2 pints) Malaga
wine or port
25 g (1 oz) split vanilla
pods

50 g (2 oz) cinnamon sticks
25 g (1 oz) ginseng root
25 g (1 oz) rhubarb

Add everything to the wine and leave to stand for five weeks. Take a small glass twice a day if suffering from flu, fatigue or depression.

Spicy Chocolate

Per person
300 ml (½ pint) milk
25 g (1 oz) plain dark
chocolate

1 slice root ginger
1 small stick of cinnamon
Honey to taste

Melt the dark chocolate in the milk in a saucepan, add the ginger and cinnamon, and simmer gently for 12 minutes. Strain and serve hot, with honey to taste.

This is one of my grandmother's recipes and she would make it if anyone had a cold. It is a delicious drink for children, and is lovely served with hot toast.

CHAPTER EIGHT

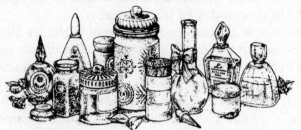

Perfumes and Flowers

Mention the word 'perfume' and the image that usually springs to mind is that of a small, exquisitely formed glass bottle filled with a luxuriously expensive liquid. For today, both men and women tend to look upon perfume purely as a form of adornment, rather like jewellery or clothes, which perhaps ought to be reserved for special occasions. But this has not always been the case. In the past, as has already been explained, there were numerous other reasons why perfumes were used and held in high esteem.

PERFUMES IN HISTORY

The word perfume derives from the Latin words for 'through smoke', and refers to the time when barks such as cinnamon and woods such as sandalwood were burned so that they gave off fumes which scented the air – a far cry from the bottled varieties with which we spray ourselves today. And looking back through history, it is clear that many of the great civilisations also used different perfumes as a means of expressing their desires or thoughts, so that they formed a sort of invisible means of communication.

I discovered that in Japan a different aromatic substance was burned at each hour of the day. It might have been citrus fruit first thing in the morning or jasmine in the afternoon, which meant that it was almost literally possible to tell the time of day by its perfume.

Similarly, in ancient Egypt, different perfumes filled the air throughout the day, but they were specifically used in order to please the sun god, Ra. At sunrise sweet resins rose to the sky to greet him from the temples where they were burned, and were replaced at midday by myrrh. Then at sunset a mixture of about sixteen different aromatic essences including frankincense expressed gratitude for his benevolence. I like the idea of Egyptians recognising the smell of sunset and knowing that as the day was closing, it was time to stop work and join together to pray and share a meal.

The Egyptian high priests were also master perfumers, whose skill in blending together different aromatic substances was highly developed. The perfumes they created were gifts to please the pharaohs, and were also burned in the temples during religious ceremonies. This was not done simply to create a pleasant aroma for the worshippers; they knew that certain aromatic substances possessed the power to influence the psyche and state of mind. They used the same skills in spiritual healing, treating people suffering from depression, anxiety and other emotional disturbances with specially prepared perfumes.

They discovered for themselves that different blends of aromatic essences could help them attain a meditative state characterised by the shifting from one plane of consciousness to another. They also believed that certain essences would cleanse the soul and bring to them a greater sense of spiritual awareness. For the worshippers, such aromas must have instilled in them feelings of blissful peace, tranquillity and detachment from reality, a state exceedingly conducive to prayer. It is also conceivable that the sight of the vapours spiralling upwards to the heavens made them feel they were forming an ephemeral link with the gods.

The Egyptians passed on their knowledge of perfumery to the Hebrew slaves, and in the Book of Exodus, when God told Moses to flee from Egypt. He reminded him to take myrrh, cinnamon, olive oil and bulrushes with him. This was so that when Moses reached his destination, and had set up God's tabernacle, he could scent it with substances that would create a spiritual atmosphere reminiscent of Egypt.

Throughout history perfumes have played a significant role in many forms of religion. In India many old temples are built of sandalwood, and its soothing fragrance is always present in the air. In some temples the practice still exists of covering the body with pure essences of rose, sandalwood, jasmine and narcissus in preparation for prayer. And in the western world, even today, incense is burned during services in churches, although most worshippers are probably ignorant of its significance.

Apart from religious and spiritual uses, however, perfumes were also used and enjoyed for the pleasure they gave to the nose. Whether the secret of a single flower or a complex mix of different aromatic essences, perfumes were used by lovers to heighten the forces of attraction that existed between them. It is said that when Cleopatra first met Antony, she ordered that her bedroom be carpeted an inch deep in fresh rose petals.

I discovered that in ancient Greece there came a time when the use of aromatics as perfumes in public places and in homes got so out of hand that the Athenian statesman Solon had to ban their sale. This was because the multi-perfumed air in Athens caused distractions through loss of concentration, and promoted allergies.

By the time Europeans eventually started taking an interest in perfume, it was probably because it was a means of suppressing the unpleasant odours that filled the air, above all else. Although the Romans had undoubtedly brought aromatic substances with them on their extensive conquests, the first mention of the use of perfume in France does not appear until the year 1190. The king at that time, Philip Augustus, bestowed upon the perfumers the privilege of exercising their skills. However, before they could do so, would-be perfumers had to practise blending aromatic essences and learn their properties, for four years; at the end of this time they had to go in front of a jury who would test their skill and knowledge.

A rather charming story tells how a special perfume was made for Queen Elizabeth of Hungary, from the essence of rosemary. Although she was eighty-one at the time, when the King of Poland met her he was so entranced by her beautiful fragrance that he asked her to marry him. It is also said that she had suffered from rheumatism until she began using the perfume; thereafter she became quite fit again.

In England, the idea of perfumery did not really catch on until the time of Elizabeth I. So delighted was she by the perfumed gloves and other scented fineries brought her by the nobleman Edward de Vere that she instructed the ladies of her court to learn the art of making aromatic waters to wear and pot-pourri to scent the rooms. Special gardens were cultivated for this purpose and a room was given to the ladies where they could create their perfumed preparations. It was during Elizabeth's reign that the ladies of the court began sewing sachets of flower petals such as rose and lavender into the seams of their voluminous skirts so that, as they swirled, scent filled the air.

Under the Queen's sympathetic eye, the perfume industry began to flourish in England, and the finest quality perfumes were to be bought, apparently, in Bucklesberry Street, London. It is said, too, that Shakespeare loved aromatic waters, and held the view that if a man wished to seduce a woman, he should always wear a perfume of civet, the acrid secretion of the wild cat.

Later, when Charles II was on the throne, a well-known and respected perfumer called Charles Lily wrote a book in which he spelled out the delights of fragrance. It was around this time that perfumes began to be used, not just for their therapeutic effects. In 1665, it was recommended that aromatic substances should be burned in every house to fight the epidemic of plague. Much later, in 1760 when George III came to power, he forbade the use of perfumes (and many other cosmetic fineries) because they were used so lavishly by whores; he even went so far as to proclaim that women who attempted to seduce men by such means would be condemned to jail for practising sorcery. This perhaps partly explains why Englishwomen chose to wear very discreet perfumes, usually single florals such as rose and lavender, for many years after!

PERFUMES TODAY

The practice of making perfumes for pleasure has reached a peak of sophistication in the twentieth century. The perfumer – known as the 'nose' – has at his disposal 2,000 aromatic substances which he can mix together in an infinite number of ways. These substances may be the essential oils extracted from the leaves and flowers of plants, the resins and barks of trees, the glandular secretions of animals such as the Abyssinian civet, the Canadian beaver, the Tibetan musk deer, and the Cachelot whale or, more commonly nowadays, chemically synthesised imitations of these aromatics. So highly trained is the nose's sense of smell that he can recognise and identify about half of all the known aromatic ingredients. (To gauge the acuity of your own sense of smell – and you'll be surprised how *difficult* it is – try the test on page 167.)

The perfumer's art is in a number of ways very similar to that of a painter or composer of music. The perfumer

Guerlain, in love with a Japanese girl, created from her the well-known Mitsouko: in it he brought together all the elements which represented that love to him, thus creating an individual 'picture' in perfume. And, just as a painter or composer can conjure up memorable scenes or events in colours or chords, the 'nose' attempts to recapture an atmosphere by recreating its smell.

I, for instance, will never forget visiting Malaysia for the first time. I was awestruck by the perfume that hung in the air, for it was an exotic mix of spicy essences such as cinnamon, nutmeg and clove and other notes contributed by durians, mangosteens, papayas and bananas, etc., all being sold in the open-air markets. The damp and humid air of the tropics − always referred to in novels as being characterised by perfumes and scents − is particularly suitable for the dispersal of odoriferous molecules. It was quite an experience for an aromatherapist, and one I shall never forget. A perfume made by mixing together those different ingredients would always conjure up an image of that visit in my mind.

(But coming back to the UK through London Airport quickly banished any such olfactory reminiscences, for I was met by the smell of commercial antiseptic! As first visual impressions are vital so, I think, are first *smell* impressions: it would be so much more pleasant to welcome visitors to this country with the smell of cloves, for clove oil, even diluted, is a very effective antiseptic. Similarly, hospital patients would be very much more relaxed if hospital cleaners used less strident antiseptics.)

When a perfumer creates a fragrance, he will use aromatic substances which will form the top notes, modifiers and base notes of the perfume. The top notes are light and volatile essences, usually of a citrus or floral nature, and responsible for the first impression a perfume gives. After a while the modifiers or middle notes, which form the heart of the perfume, will come through; these are often essences like rose and jasmine. They are supported by the rich, lingering base notes, such as sandalwood, oakmoss, musk or civet.

In this way, the character of the perfume, created by the interplay between the various different essences, slowly reveals itself and its personality. For a perfume *does* have its own personality. It may be fresh and mischievous, rich and provocative, or heady and seductive – the possibilities are endless due to the multitude of ways in which different aromatic substances can be blended together.

Another interesting phenomenon about a perfume is that it will never smell exactly the same on any two individuals. This is because each person has their own body fragrance, created by their pheromones, and this interacts with the notes in the perfume to modify or alter its aroma. For this reason it is never a good idea to choose a perfume on the grounds that it smelled wonderful on your friend; it will smell different on you. You may also find that because the quality of pheromones is affected by physical and emotional changes taking place in the body, a perfume may smell heavenly one day, and very disappointing the next.

When buying a perfume for the first time, it is vital to go alone, and in good mental and physical health. A friend might influence you, literally or subconsciously, and the different pheromones emitted when, say, depressed or unwell, would change the smell of the perfume on your skin. Try a drop or two on your wrist, and don't smell it from too near or your nose will be 'blinded'; hold your wrist at a reasonable distance, and waft it about to allow the odoriferous molecules to rise naturally, Leave for at least two hours, and then 'see' how the perfume has changed or matured. Then, if you still like it, go back and buy the perfume, but not until the next day, just to make sure!

You don't have to stick to one perfume either. As your

moods change, as your social personality changes – at work or out dancing for instance – you may want to wear a different perfume. It is quite fascinating to me that so many women like to possess a number of different perfumes, presumably to suit the different facets of their personality, while men will usually remain loyal to just one aftershave.

Perfume is much more than mere decorative frivolity. It can and should be an extension of your personality, for together with the way you dress, it reinforces the image you have of yourself, and provides another outlet for communicating it to others. Perfume can also be a master of illusions, for it can lend a hint of flamboyance to someone usually rather shy or reserved, a flamboyance which may only be detected through the nose. Carnation, for instance, is known for its ability to banish shyness and induce courage, and I always dab a little essential oil on my chest before I have to speak in front of an audience (in fact, French criminals are said to wear a carnation in their buttonholes for a day before a big job, in order to build up their aggression and nerve!).

But you should always beware of wearing *too* much perfume. It's generally thought of as a little vulgar, but it also makes you appear rather aggressive – which of course the perfume itself *is* if in too great a quantity. So, if you are meeting someone important (unless you *want* to intimidate), apply perfume discreetly and modestly.

Perfumes, like all smells, leave strong impressions on the subconscious mind, and the memory of a person, or indeed of a place, is almost always influenced by the aromatic vapours present at the time. A supernatural hint of this is contained in the intriguing story told me by a man about his mother. One day he became very aware of the perfume his mother always used in the air; in fact it seemed to follow him wherever he went. Not having seen his mother for some time, he could not understand the meaning of this phenomenon until he heard, the next day, that his mother had died the day before.

PERFUMES AND THE PSYCHE

As the Egyptians discovered so many years ago, perfumes can profoundly affect a person's emotional and mental state. This is not, however, true of most of today's commercial perfumes for they contain chemically synthesised aromatics which do not possess the same therapeutic properties as their natural counterparts. Natural perfumes also have the advantage of being kind to the olfactory organ, not like some of the rather overpowering, cloying synthetic ones which can actually make you feel ill.

The Greek physician Hippocrates – 'the father of medicine' – said: 'The way to health is to have an aromatic bath and scented massage every day.' He knew that good health embodies both a healthy body and a healthy mind – the two are inseparable. He was aware, as were the Egyptians, that essential oils could influence the psyche and benefit the state of mind. When I was in Paris I attended a lecture on aromatherapy given by an Indian doctor called Badmajieff. He echoed Hippocrates when he said: 'Odoriferous molecules can influence a person's emotions, mental state and philosophy. The way of life is through the essential oils of plants.'

How essential oils work in this way has only emerged in recent years. As said before, the nerves of the olfactory organ are linked to the limbic portion of the brain responsible, amongst other things, for modifying emotional well-being. This is why pleasant smells make us feel happy while noxious smells make us depressed and irritable.

Certain essential oils also have a beneficial action on the nervous system. In times of stress the sympathetic branch of the nervous system becomes dominant, and if such a situation is prolonged, you become tired, thoughts are shattered and everyday problems grow out of proportion. Essential oils work to re-establish the equilibrium between the sympathetic and the para-sympathetic branches of the nervous system and in doing so not only relax the body, but also restore clarity to the mind, stimulate the thought processes, and bring back lost feelings of awareness and control.

Most essences are stimulants. They galvanise the adrenal cortex into action, which leaves you better able to cope with stress than might have been possible before. Stress, as is well known, is a major cause of anxiety, depression, irritability, nervousness, insomnia and even lack of interest in sex.

Indeed certain essential oils have long been praised for their aphrodisiac properties. One of the reasons why they work so fast and effectively is because again they act directly on the limbic portion of the brain, which is also responsible for modulating sexual behaviour. So, it would seem that Cleopatra's rose petals were sensible quite apart from being romantic!

In a rather less direct way, other essences possess the ability to dynamise fatigued reproductive glands into action, and so work to revive a waning interest in sex.

So whenever you make a perfume composed of one or more essential oils you must ask yourself what kind of function you wish it to perform as well as how you want it to smell. As perfumes, the following essential oils can be added to the bath, or to some oil and massaged into the skin. You could also place a few drops on a glass slide and leave it near a radiator or light so their vapours fill the air, or take them internally in the form of herb teas.

Aphrodisiac

Most effective: cinnamon, savory, ylang ylang, sage, ginger, and rose.

Others: anise, fennel, clove, marjoram, mint, nutmeg, rosemary, vervain, neroli.

Anxiety (effective against)

Most effective: basil, marjoram.
Others: coriander, tarragon, fennel, hyssop, lavender, mint, orange, rosemary, thyme and vervain.

Nightmare (to banish)

Most effective: basil, lemon, fennel, mint, rosemary.
Others: marjoram, orange, sage.

Insomnia (to treat)

Most effective: basil, camomile, lavender, melissa, mandarin, orange, neroli, rosemary, thyme, rose.

Depression (to relieve)

Angelica, basil, carrot, lemon, coriander, ginger, eucalyptus, lavender, mandarin, marjoram, melissa, mint, neroli and parsley.

Exercise (to prime the body for action, aid perspiration and encourage deep breathing)

Most effective: rosemary, ylang ylang, eucalyptus, benzoin.
Others: cardamom, mint, carnation, angelica, galbanum.

Concentration (to help you study)

Carnation, coriander, rosemary, basil, bergamot.

THE LANGUAGE OF FLOWERS

Our ancestors undoubtedly attached far greater meaning to flowers than we do today. The Egyptians and the Chinese used them as a mean of communicating messages to one another, and many years later, the Victorians used flowers to express different sentiments. A few of their ideas linger today – we still send red roses to someone we love – but most have long been forgotten.

I think it would be a nice idea to start using flower language again, so I list some of the flowers and their meanings below.

Red roses	Passion
White roses	Spiritual love
Yellow roses	Infidelity
Anemones	Refusal
Azalea	Passion
Bramble	Envy
Foxglove	Insincerity
Heliotrope	Devoted attachment
Gardenia	Secret love
Ivy	Fidelity, and confiding love
Jasmine	Joy and passion
Lemon blossom	Fidelity
Lilac	New love
Lily of the valley	Happiness

But we could also extend this language, by using the aroma of flowers to create atmosphere, to cure or heal, or to achieve a required result.

On the first of May in France, for instance, friends and member of the family will give each other bunches and bowls of lily of the valley, presumably to wish each other happiness. But lily of the valley has another effect as well. My grandmother, who had a mild heart condition, always amused us by claiming that the perfume of lily of the valley made her feel better, that her palpitations were lessened, and that she didn't feel so dizzy. She planted many in her garden, near to the windows of the house, and would have bowls of the flowers near where she was sitting or working. It wasn't until years later that I discovered that lily of the valley does actually possess a substance which is used in the treatment of heart conditions by many French herbalists. You could grow the flowers near the house, cut them for inside use, and dry them, to use them in this way.

And flowers do not have to be a gift to be romantic. To create a romantic atmosphere at home, use and arrange those flowers associated with love or passion – or their essences – and perfume the bedroom (like Cleopatra) with roses, jasmine or gardenia. If cooking for a lover, serve a light meal (the rice cake on page 145 with added ginseng is a nourishing and effective aphrodisiac), and don't allow too highly perfumed flowers on the table to clash with your aromatic food.

THE PERFUMED GARDEN

It was during the reign of Elizabeth I that flowers and herbs for gardens were chosen not only for their aesthetic value but also for their perfumes and therapeutic properties. Indeed, Elizabethan England became renowned for its beautifully fragrant and romantic gardens – tended on the whole by the women, while the men saw to the vegetables. The poet Francis Bacon wrote of such gardens: 'Those which perfume the air most delightfully not passed by as the rest, but being trodden upon and crushed are three, that is burnet, wild thyme and watermints. Therefore, you are to set whole alleys of them to have the pleasure when you walk or tread.'

I do not profess to be a skilled gardener, but the fragrance of the different flowers, trees, shrubs and herbs and their curative properties are, for me, far more valuable than their colours and shapes. I think it important that the notes of each aromatic plant harmonise as they do in a perfume; and that they should be mentally uplifting, so that walking in the garden will always be a pleasurable experience to the nose.

Once you have a knowledge of the properties of the various aromatic essences, you will be able to choose the plants for your garden to suit your desires and needs. I am merely going to give a few tips on which plants are companionable, which are not, and where each one belongs in your perfumed garden.

Medicinal plants like camomile, basil, calendula, hyssop, hops, mint, sage, fennel and lemon verbena should form the heart of your fragrant garden. They may be surrounded by shrubs of rosemary, thyme and the evergreen sweet bay, for these plants seal in the perfume which radiates from the medicinals. Lavender is perfect for planting along either side of a path, and behind this sweet-smelling shrub, damask roses and centifolia roses smell good.

Roses also go well with the citrus-like bergamot plant, and with the cooler camomile. French folklore has it that roses benefit from being interspersed with garlic, for its potent aroma keeps the greenfly and other destructive insects at bay.

Never grow carnations in the same beds as roses for they do not go well together, and produce a highly aggressive atmosphere. This applies especially to selecting flowers for perfuming your living room. When you *do* plant carnations, choose the old-fashioned varieties for they have a sweet spicy smell which is a good nerve tonic and also gives courage to shy people. For this reason, an arrangement of carnations might be a good idea in the home or office of someone wishing to be *less* shy.

For lining smaller, meandering paths, chose herbs such as mint, parsley, and chives, and if you have a garden seat, surround it with aromatic rosemary.

Angelica and artemisia also go well in a perfumed garden because they are quite fragrant, and can be planted as and where you wish. You might bed some pelargonium in a corner of your garden, for both the leaves and flowers are scented and you can detect their perfume from a distance. Camomile, lemon verbena and mint also grow well in proximity to this flower.

If you have a shady or wooded area in your garden, plant some lily of the valley for they love such conditions and have a delightful aroma too.

To seal in the perfume generated within your garden, plant pine and cypress trees at the back as they form a barrier which prevents the odoriferous molecules from escaping. They also have a beneficial action on the respiratory system, as does lilac, although it unfortunately only flowers for a short period of time.

A eucalyptus would be useful at the bottom of your garden, firstly because of its stunning silvery foliage, and secondly because it keeps the flies away during the summer months.

Train honeysuckle and jasmine to climb around your house, so that when you open the windows their fragrance seeps into the rooms. Do not have them around your bedroom, however, of if you do always close the window at night; their scents are very stimulating and will prevent you from falling asleep. A lime tree would be lovely near a bedroom window, or perhaps a few orange trees (not too common in Great Britain), because of their calming and tranquillising influence.

If you like growing your own vegetables, it might be worth considering planting marigolds with them, for their scent helps to keep the insects away. In a similar manner, mint and sage protect cabbages.

Of course, different flowers bloom at different times of the year, and some careful thought will need to go into selecting your plants so that their fragrances will mingle together at the same time.

For spring, it will be a good idea to plant daffodils, bluebells and narcissi as their perfumes all harmonise with each other. And, for the winter months, make sure you have planted plenty of hyacinths near your windows, or indoors, for their fragrance will bring untold pleasure to a grey and cloudy day.

APPENDICES

Test Your Sense of Smell

You can first *improve* your sense of smell by introducing a new smell into your life every day. It could be from flowers, fruit, vegetables, herbs or essential oils, even chemicals used in the household (the latter could be important as they will enable you to recognise the presence of dangerous toxic fumes in the home).

The way to approach new smells is to sniff or inhale the odours or scents at a distance of 5–10 cm (2–4 inches). Close your eyes and visualise the item and continue the process for as many times as you wish, until you have the smell fixed in your mind. Have a notepad nearby and make some record of your reactions to the smell. For example, whether you liked or disliked it, whether you found it hot or cold, whether it was strong or subtle, musky, floral, pepperminty, putrid, pungent, camphorous, citrus and so on. After all, this is how wine tasters, who *smell* as well as taste, develop their art; and no serious brandy drinker would taste until he had warmed the snifter and inhaled the rising fumes.

Here is a simple game to play with your family or friends, which could make an interesting alternative to 'Kim's Game' for a children's party. The first rule is that one person at a time should be blindfolded and tested on their ability to recognise ten different smells. These are listed on a notepad and the person's performance is marked against each item. The second rule is that the person being tested must not *touch* the objects which they are trying to identify. And if the other 'contestants' are in the room, the objects must be given in a different order each time. Clues to the items being smelled can be given to beginners and the winner is the one who has scored the highest marks.

Choose your odoriferous substances from anything you have available. Vegetables should be cut into to release their smell as should some fruit; other fruit, like citrus, may need their peel scraped to release their pungency, and herbs like rosemary or bay may need a preliminary squeeze.

The following lists give a selection of various testable odoriferous items to use.

Fruit

Apple
Banana
Lemon
Melon
Orange
Peach
Pineapple
Strawberry
Raspberry
Tangerine

Herbs

Basil
Bay
Dill
Fennel
Marjoram
Mint
Rosemary
Sage
Tarragon
Thyme

Store-cupboard Ingredients

Coffee
Honey
Mustard
Orange (or other) marmalade
Peanut butter
Raspberry (or other) jam
Redcurrant (or other) jelly
Spices such as cloves,
    coriander, cumin, curry
    powder, ginger, nutmeg, etc.
Tea (Indian and Chinese)
Yeast

Vegetables

Asparagus
Broccoli
Brussels sprouts
Cauliflower
Celery
Fennel
Garlic
Horseradish
Mushrooms
Onion

Fluids

Brandy
Coca-cola
Gin
Lubricating oil
Methylated spirits
Sherry
Turpentine
Vinegar
Whisky
Wine

Household Staples

Aftershave
Face cream
Firelighters
Furniture polish
Perfume
Shampoo
Shaving cream
Soap powder
Toothpaste
Washing-up liquid
Bleach

Bibliography

Bardeau, Fabric, *Le Medicine par les fleurs*, Paris, 1967

Bezanger-Beauquesne L., Pinkas M. and Torck M., *Les Plantes dans la Thérapeutique Moderne*, Paris, 1975

Bourret, Jean-Claude, *Le Défi de la Médicine par les Plantes*, Paris, 1978

Burton, Robert, *The Language of Smell*, London, 1976

Cabanes Dr., *Remèdes d'Autrefois*, Paris, 1913

Deville, Michel, *Santé et nature*, Paris, 1980

Lagriffe, Louis, *Le livre des Epices, condiments et aromates*, Paris, 1968

Leca, A. P., *La Médicine Egyptienne*, Paris, 1971

Leclerc, H., *Précis de phytothérapie*, Paris, 1976

Lehane, Brendan, *Le Pouvoir des Plantes* Paris, 1976

Marks, Ronald, *Psoriasis*, London, 1981

Maury, Marguerite, *Le Capital Jeunesse*, Paris, 1961

Morelle, Jean, *Traité de Biochimie Cutanée*, Paris, 1957

Naves, Y. R., *Technologie et Chimie des Parfums Naturels*, Paris, 1974

Valnet, Jean, *Aromathérapie*, Paris, 1975
Phytothérapie, Paris, 1979

Winter, Ruth, *Le livre des odeurs*, Paris, 1978

Index to Conditions Treated with Essential Oils

Index to Conditions Treated with Other Aromatherapeutic Substances

Index

Ordering by Post

If you fill in the form below and send it to:
Daniele Ryman Limited, Suite 101, Park Lane Hotel,
Piccadilly, London W1Y 8BX
you will receive a free brochure of all Daniele Ryman's
exciting products, from natural perfume to facial cleansers,
creams, face and body oils.

Name...

Address ....

....

....

Telephone Number...

For Readers in the U.S.A.

The American Aromatherapy Association
P.O. Box 1222
Fair Oaks
CA 95628